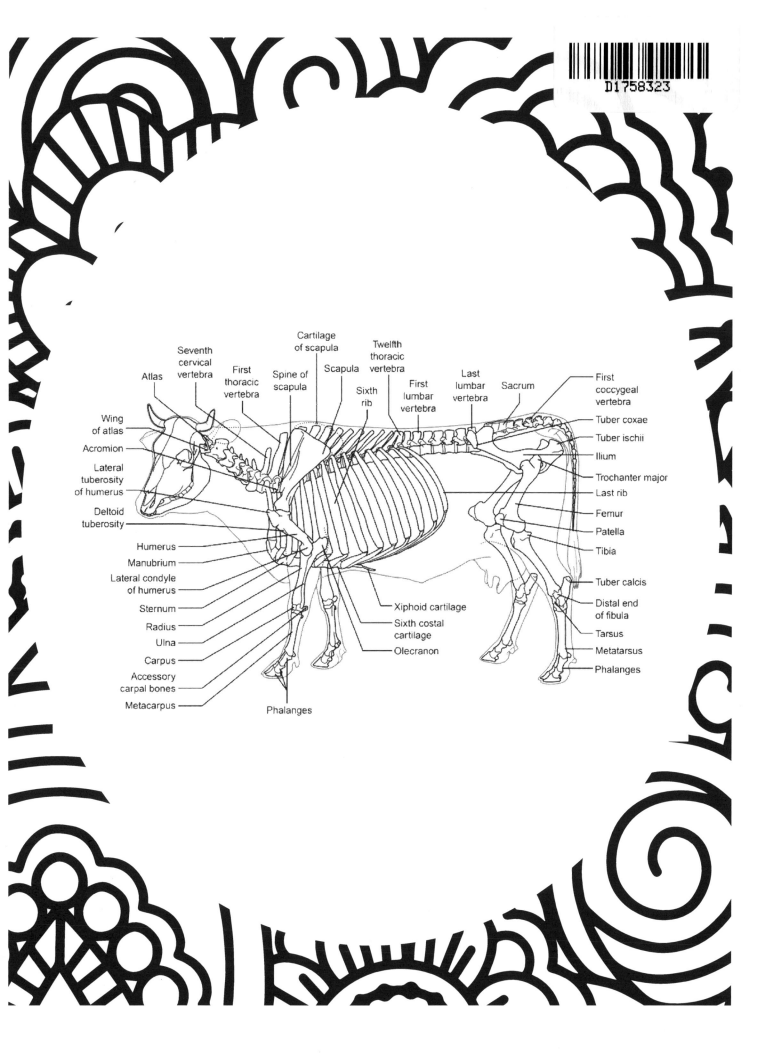

This Book Belongs To

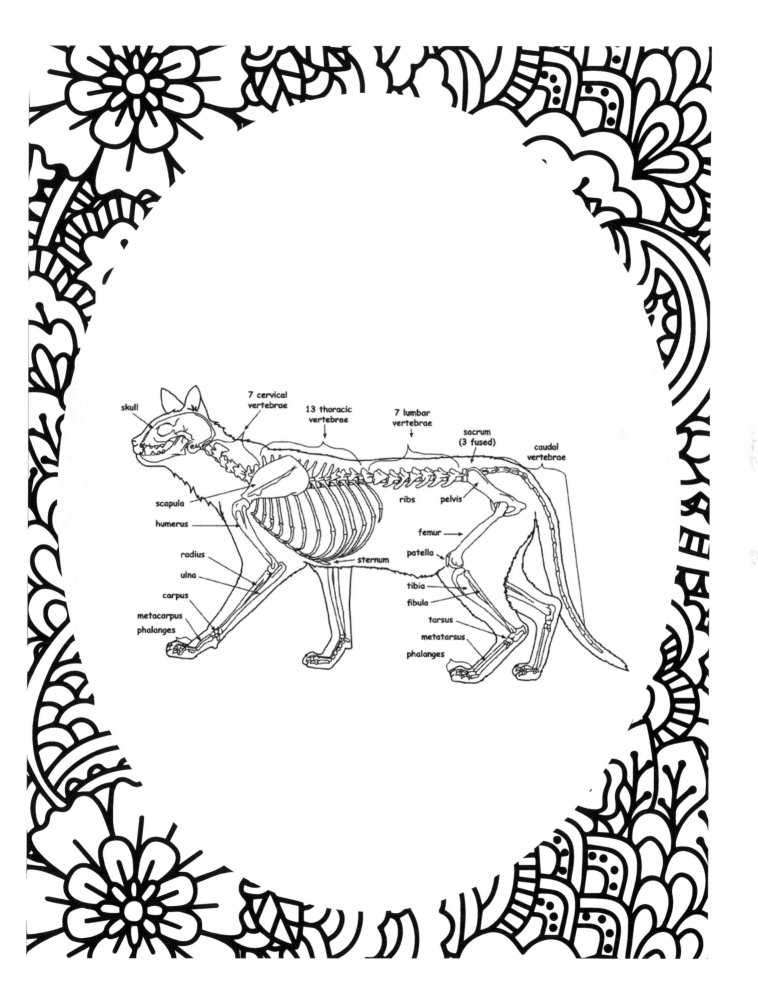

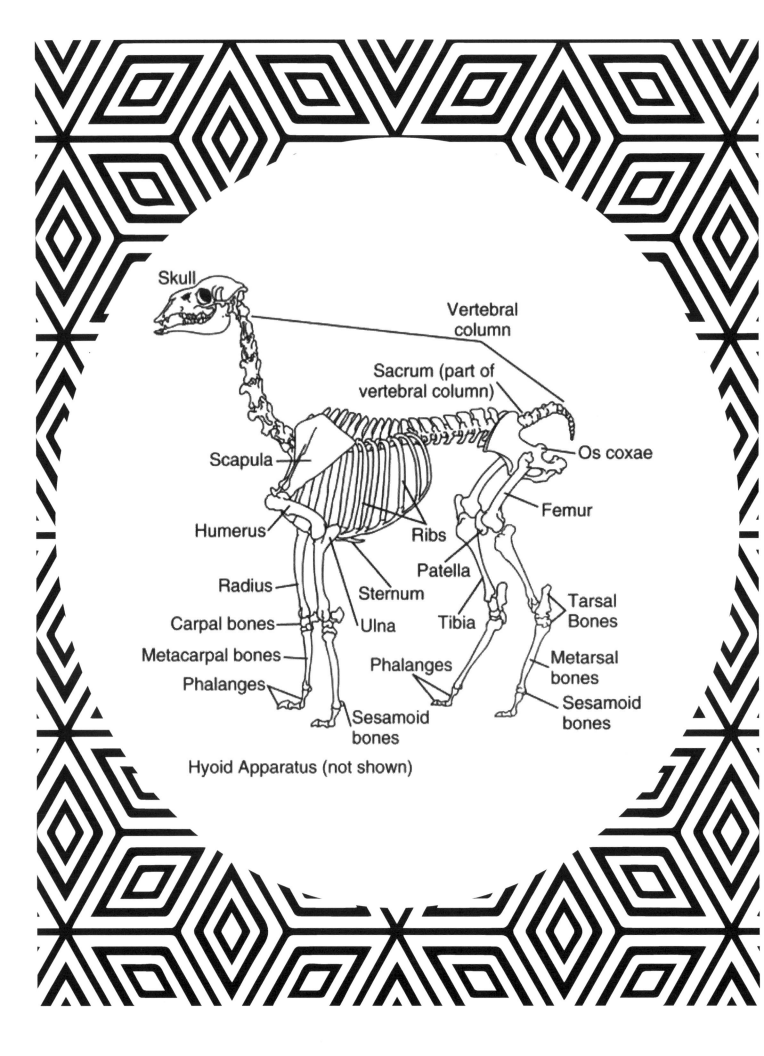

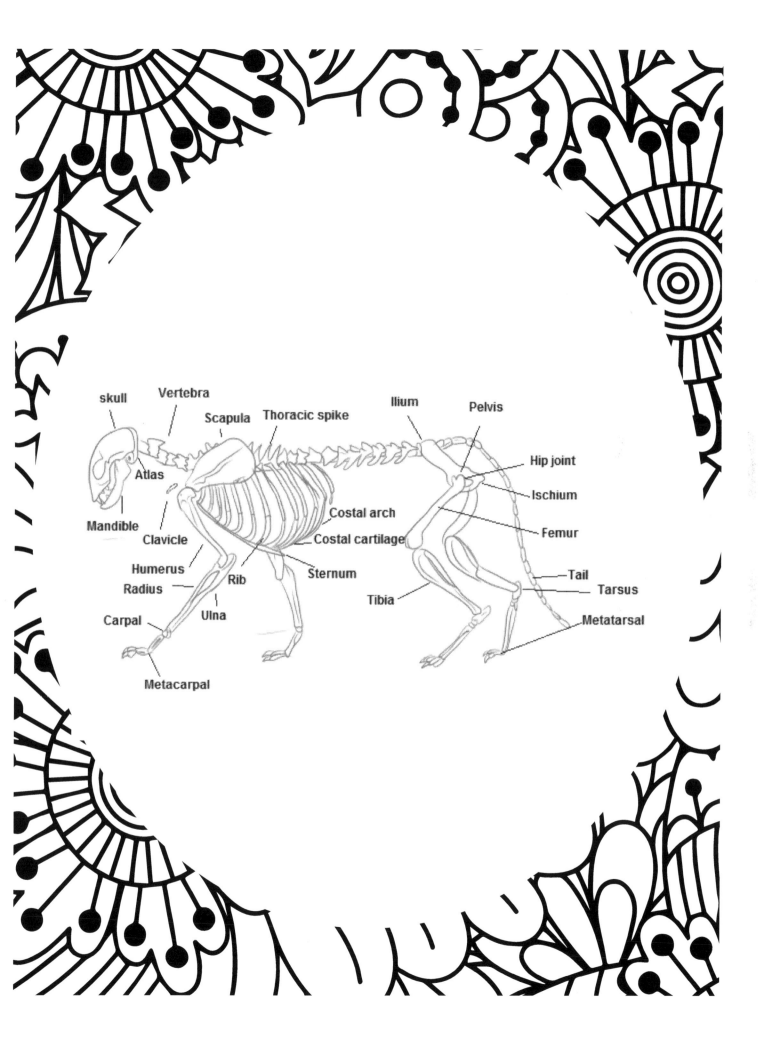

Rat

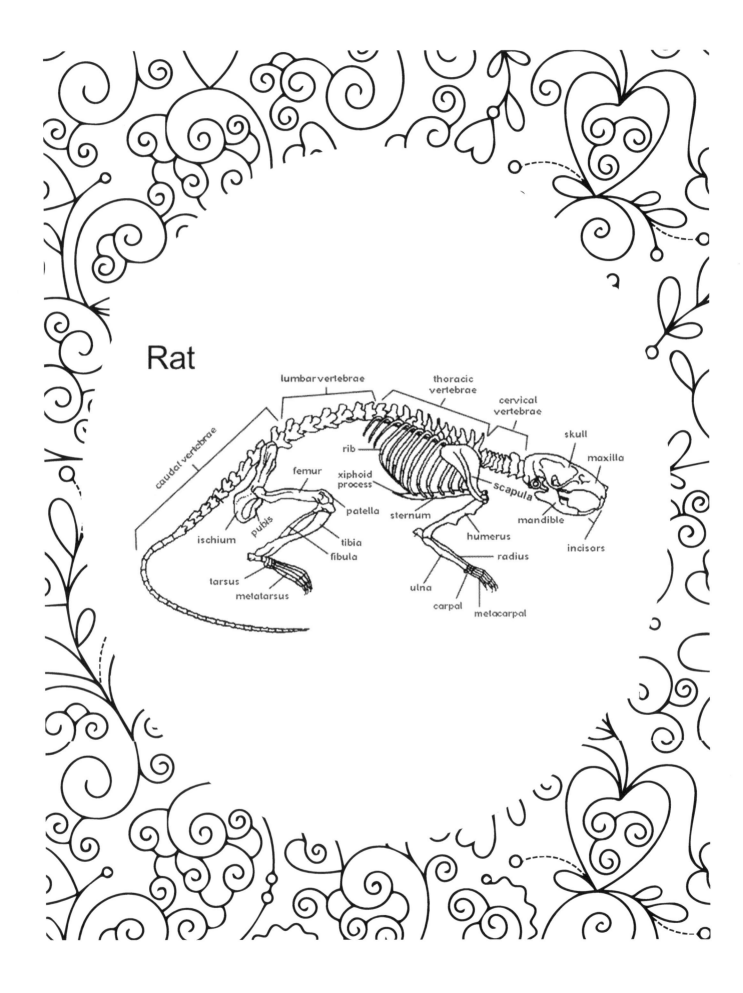

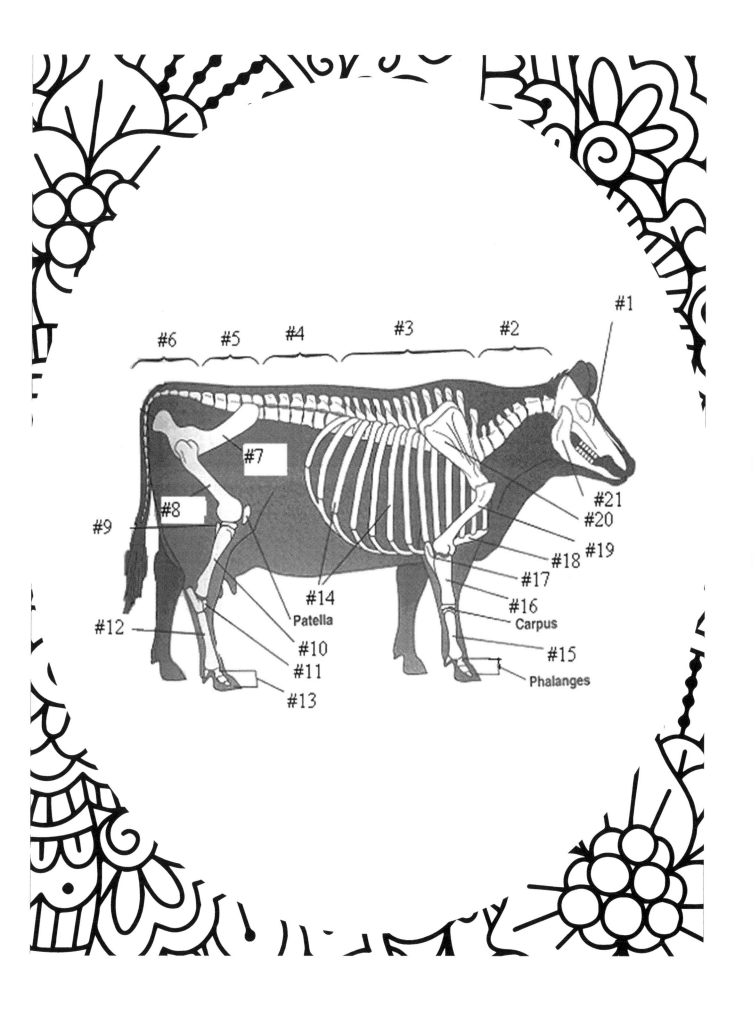

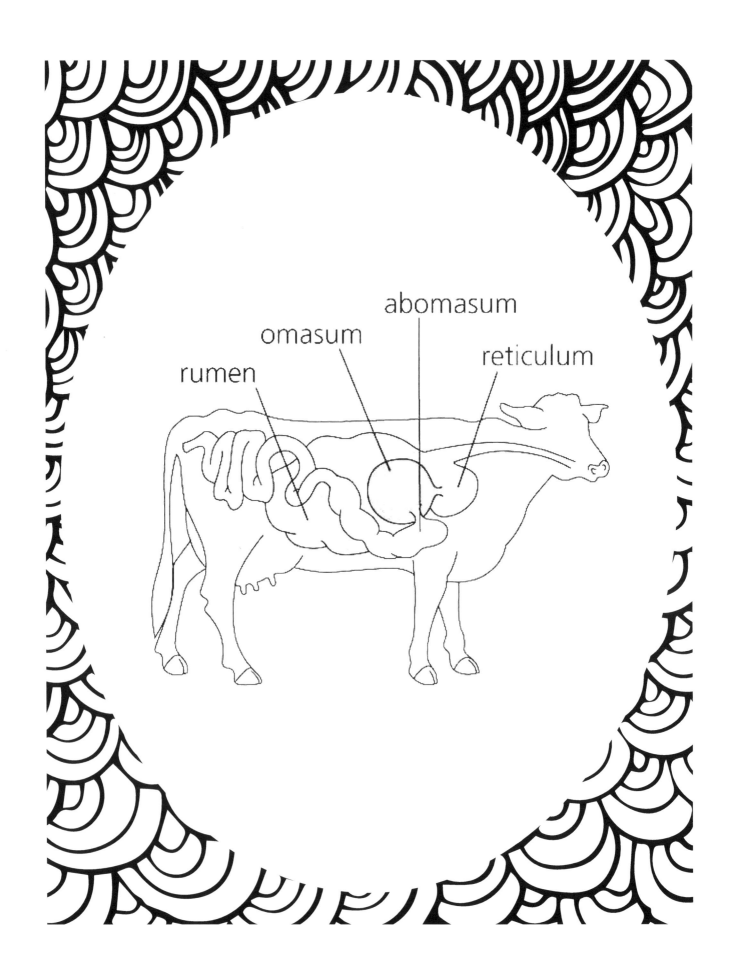

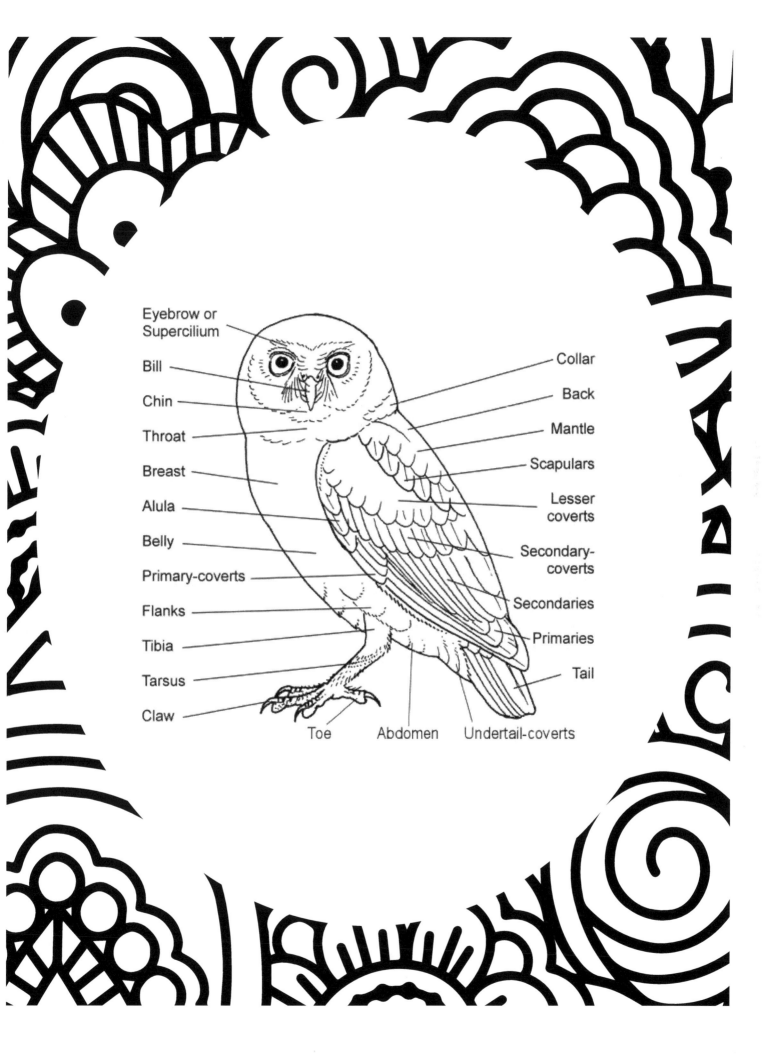

Eyebrow or Supercilium

Bill

Chin

Throat

Breast

Alula

Belly

Primary-coverts

Flanks

Tibia

Tarsus

Claw

Collar

Back

Mantle

Scapulars

Lesser coverts

Secondary-coverts

Secondaries

Primaries

Tail

Toe

Abdomen

Undertail-coverts

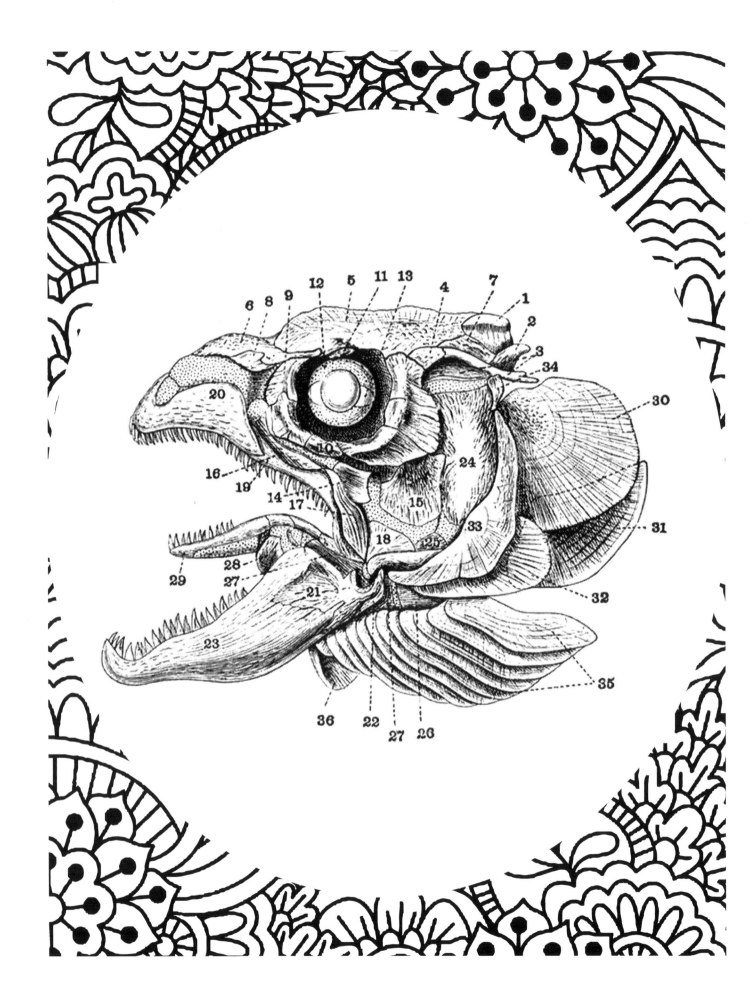

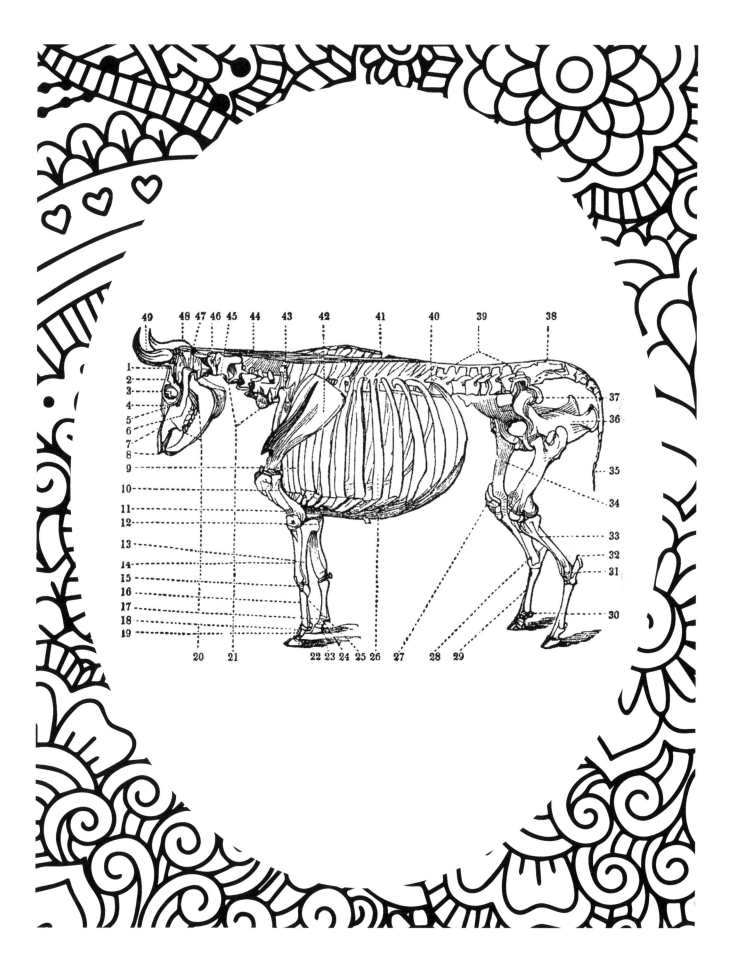

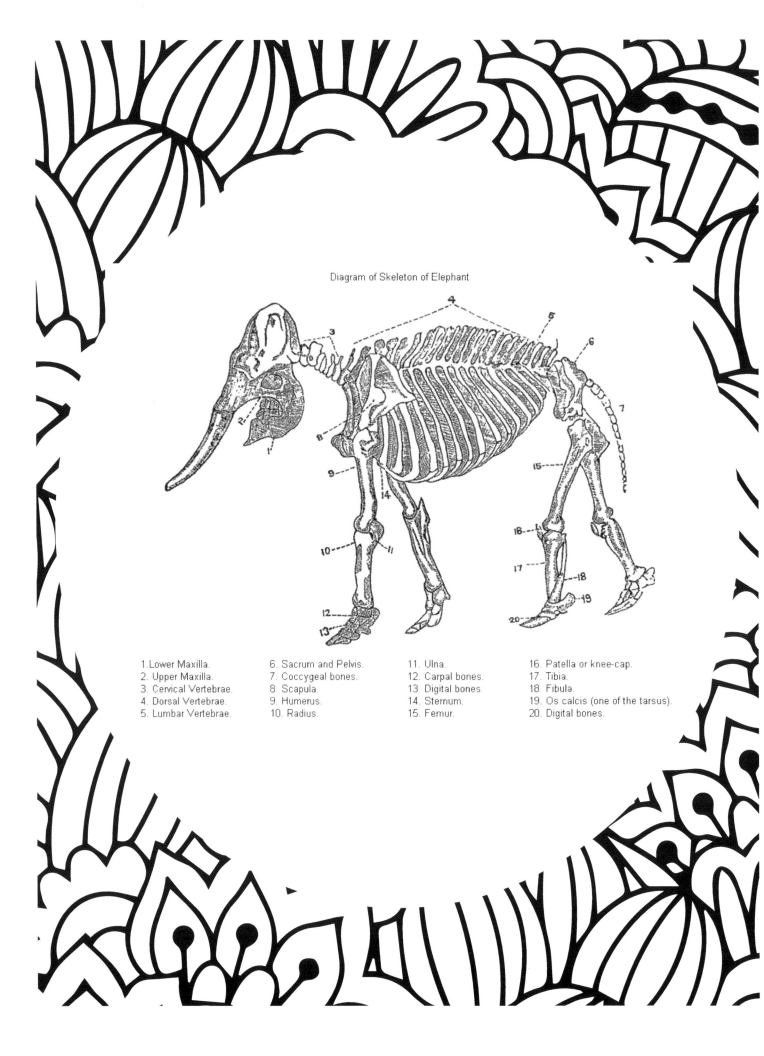

Diagram of Skeleton of Elephant

1. Lower Maxilla.
2. Upper Maxilla.
3. Cervical Vertebrae.
4. Dorsal Vertebrae.
5. Lumbar Vertebrae.
6. Sacrum and Pelvis.
7. Coccygeal bones.
8. Scapula.
9. Humerus.
10. Radius.
11. Ulna.
12. Carpal bones.
13. Digital bones
14. Sternum.
15. Femur.
16. Patella or knee-cap.
17. Tibia.
18. Fibula.
19. Os calcis (one of the tarsus).
20. Digital bones.

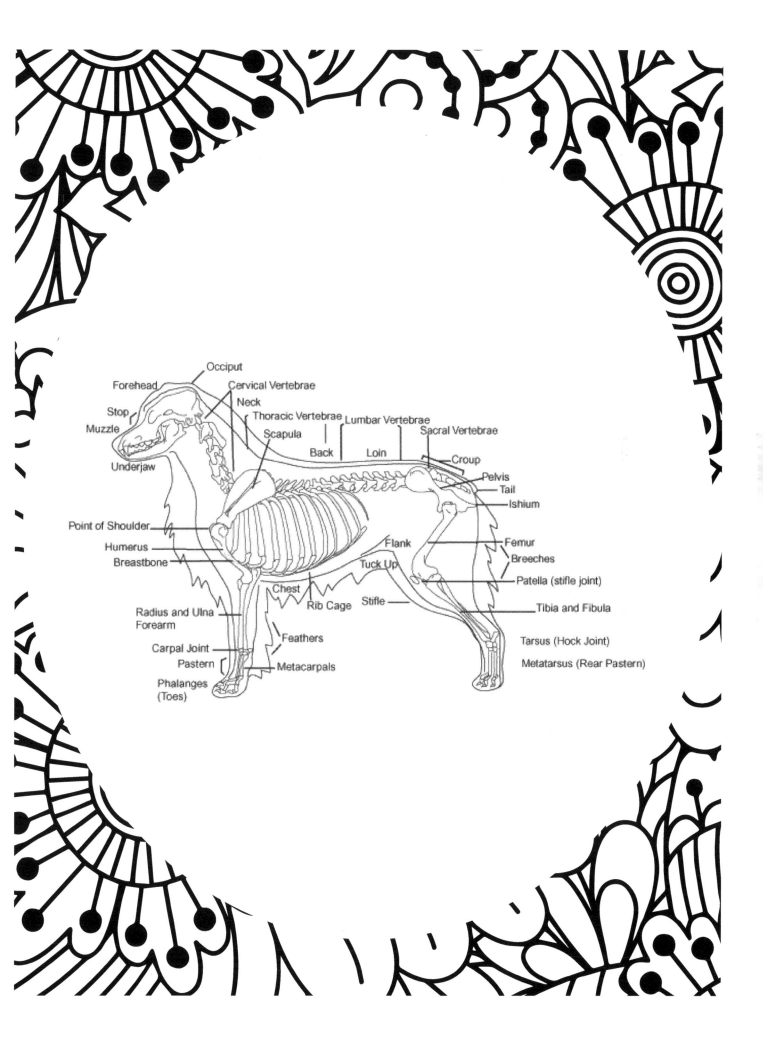

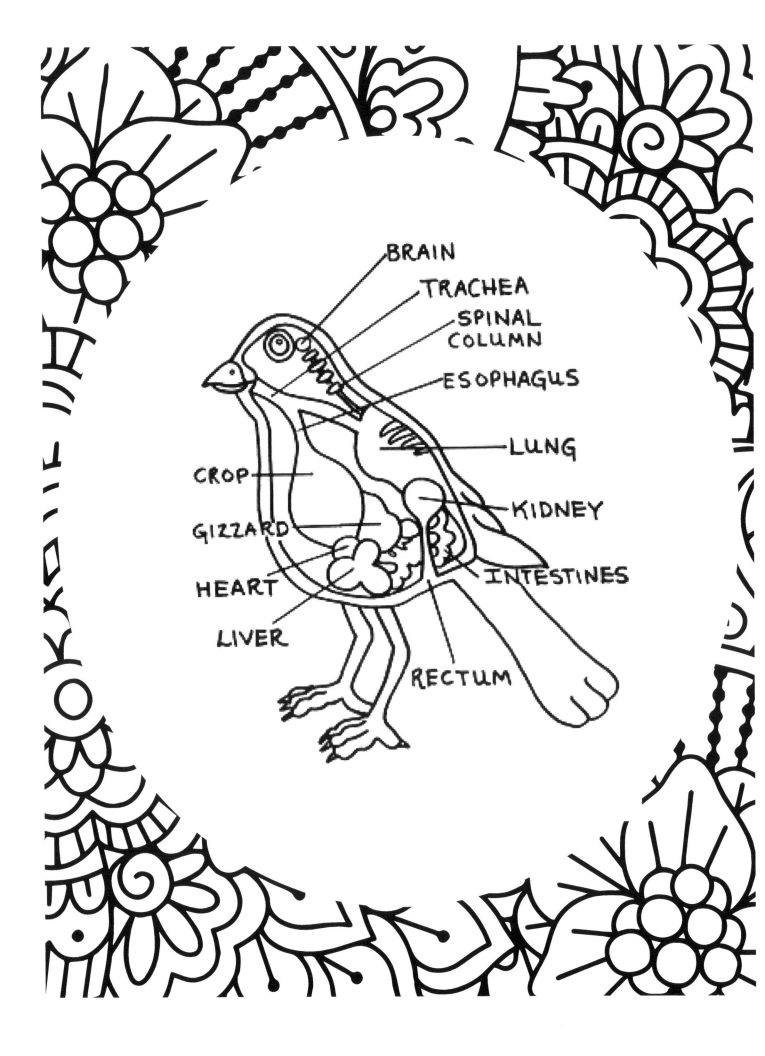

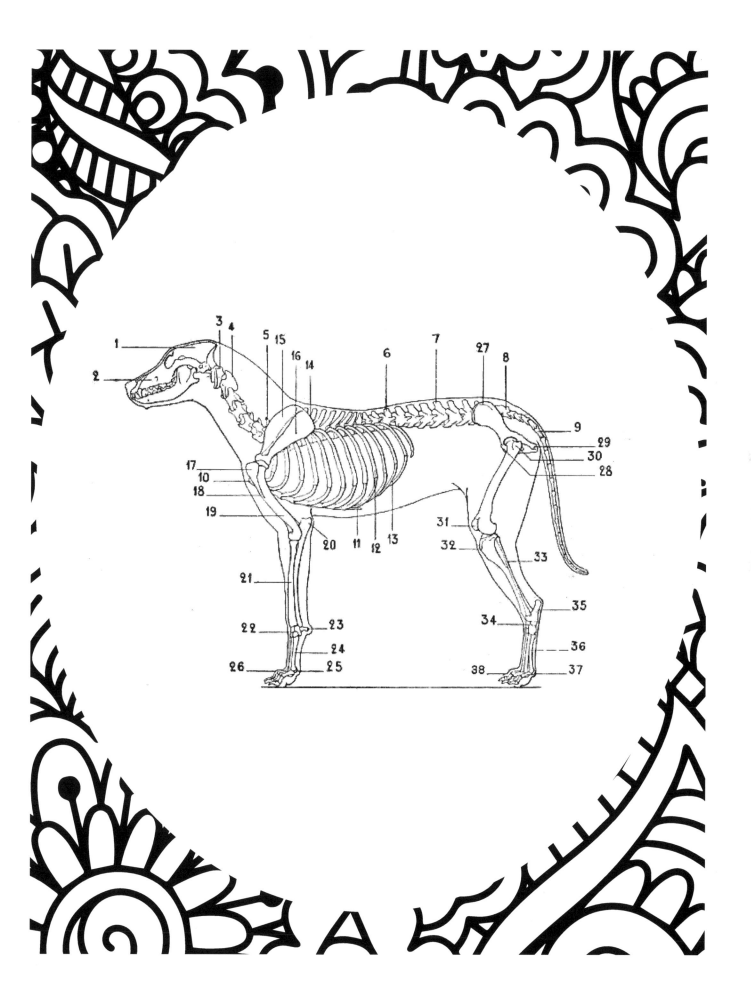

Name the Cat's Organs

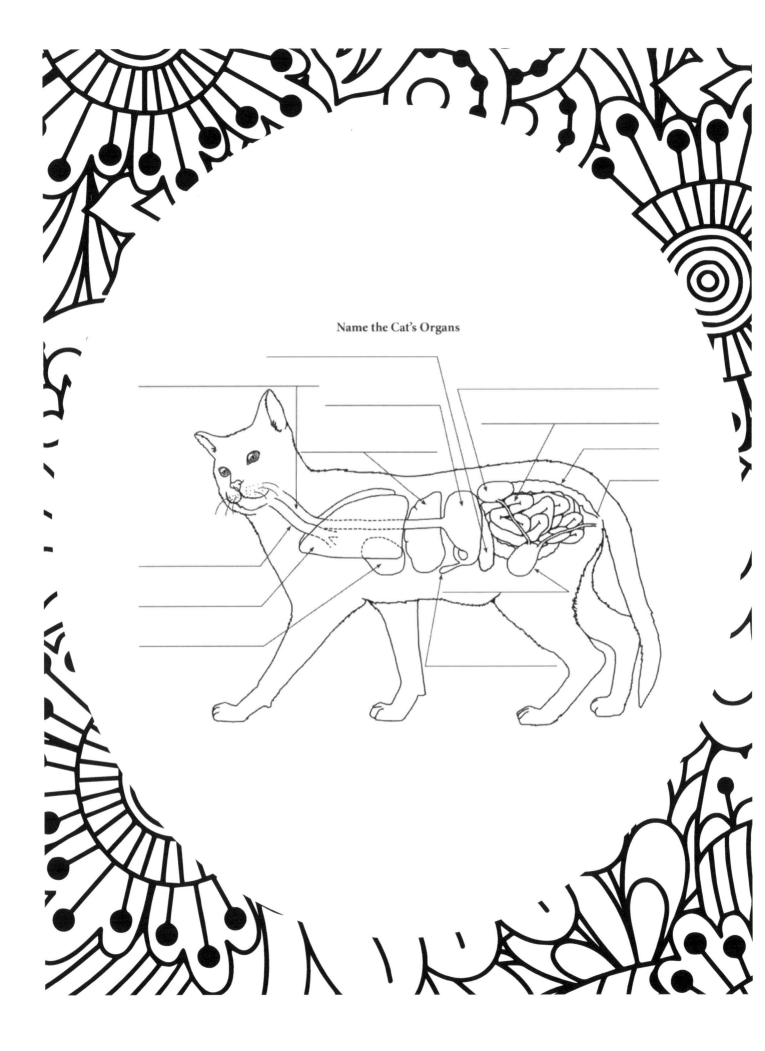

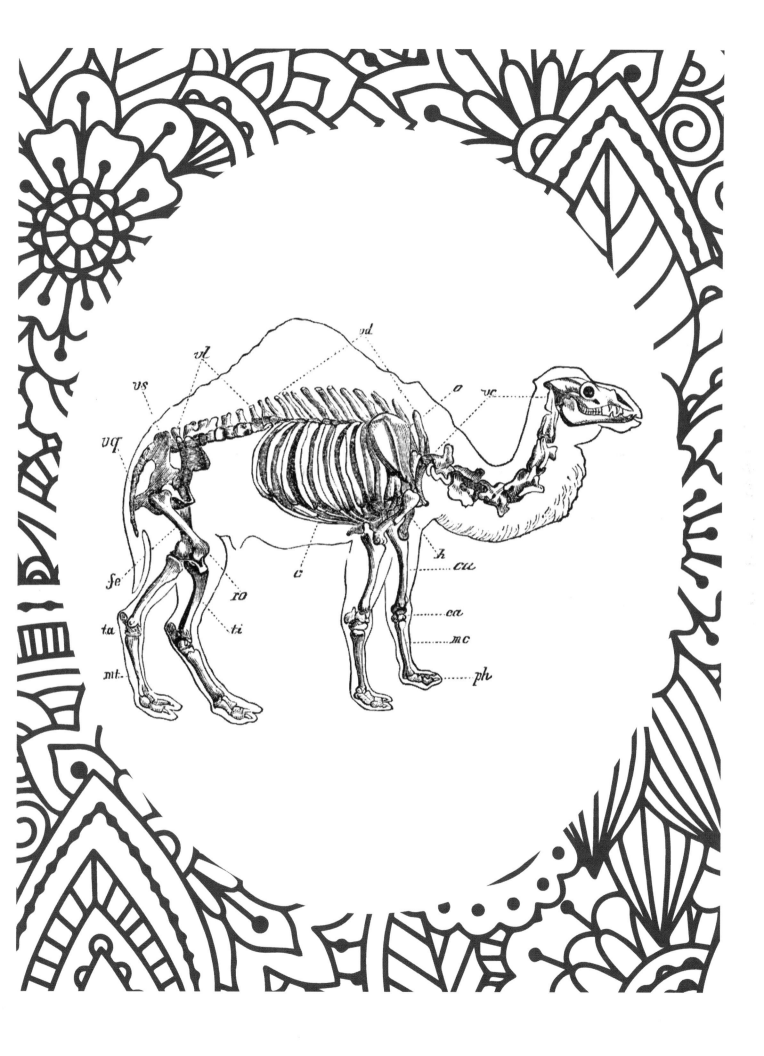

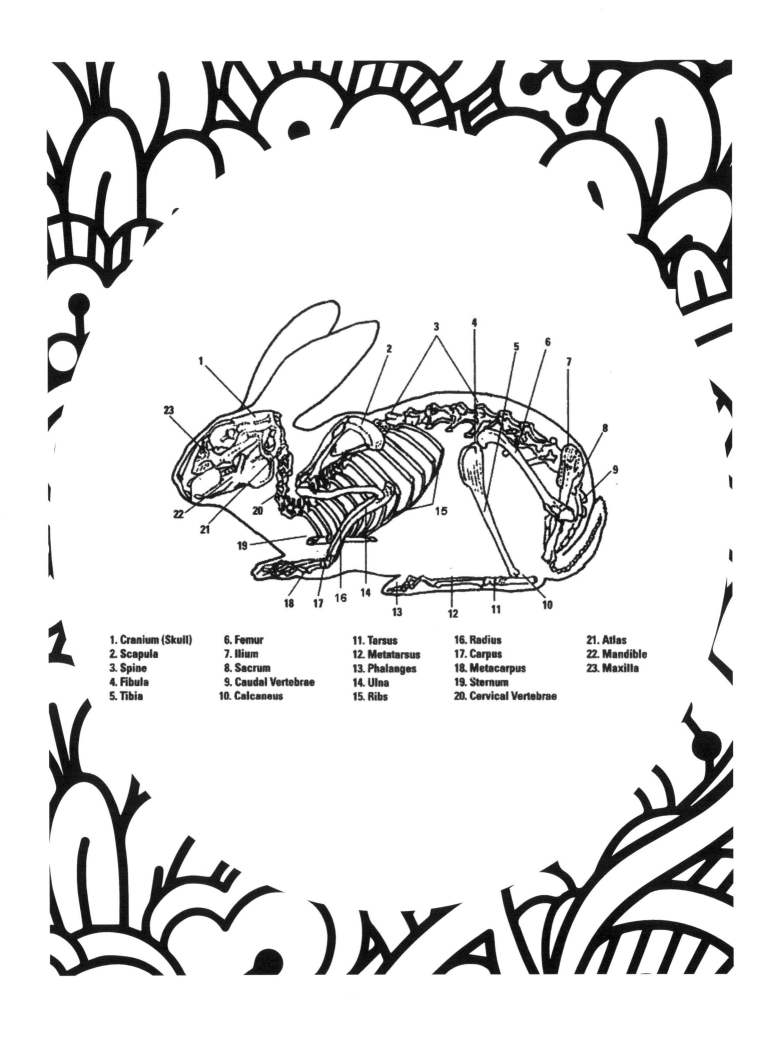

1. Cranium (Skull)
2. Scapula
3. Spine
4. Fibula
5. Tibia
6. Femur
7. Ilium
8. Sacrum
9. Caudal Vertebrae
10. Calcaneus
11. Tarsus
12. Metatarsus
13. Phalanges
14. Ulna
15. Ribs
16. Radius
17. Carpus
18. Metacarpus
19. Sternum
20. Cervical Vertebrae
21. Atlas
22. Mandible
23. Maxilla

Dinosaur osteology primer (learn the bones!)

Cervical
Vertebrae
Dorsal
Vertebrae
Sacral
Vertebrae
Caudal
Vertebrae
Skull
Ilium
Ischium
Femur
Fibula
Chevrons
Mandible
Ribs
Gastralia
Pubis
Tibia
Pes

Scapula
Furcula
Coracoid
Sternum
Manus

Humerus
Radius
Ulna
Carpal
Metacarpals
Ungual
Phalanges

Tarsals
Metatarsals
Phalanges
Ungual

Copyright Scott Hartman, 2013.

ANATOMY OF A HORSE HOOF

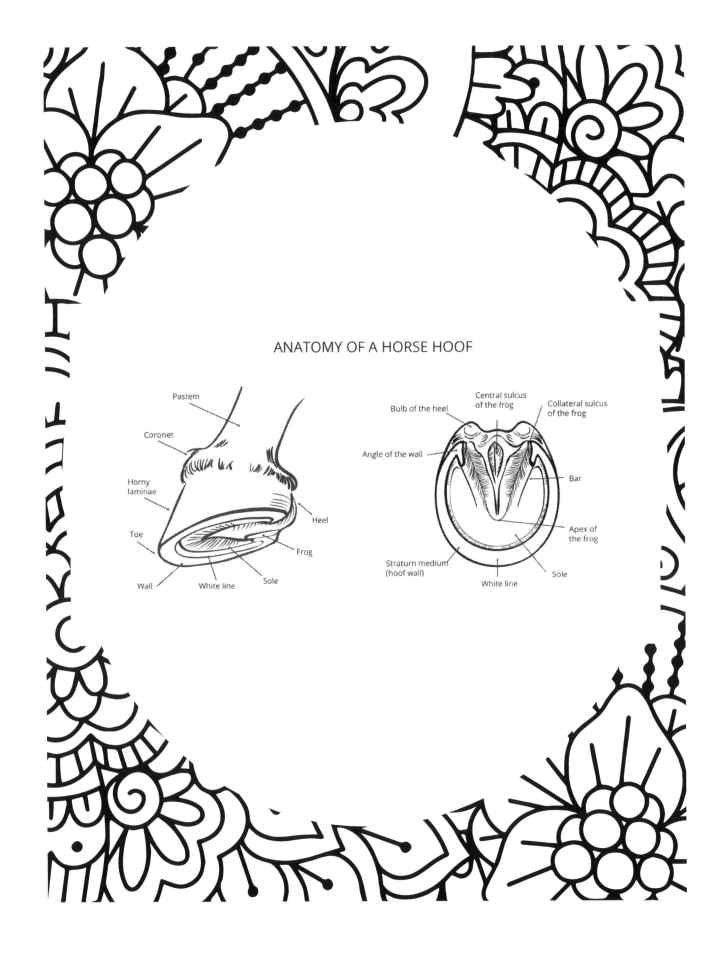

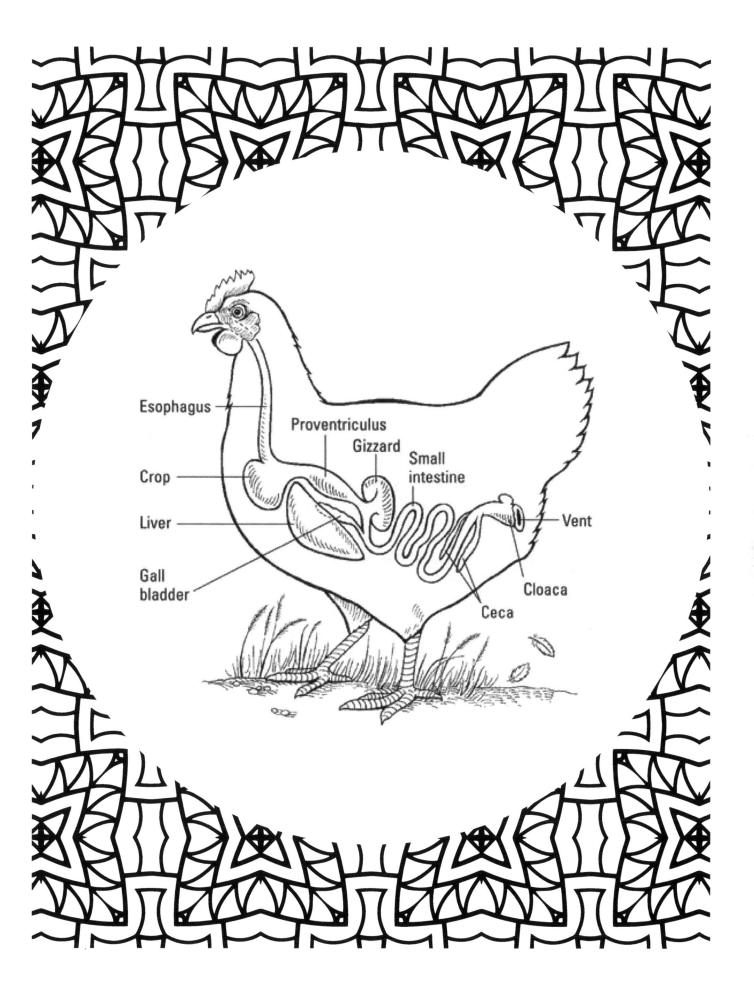

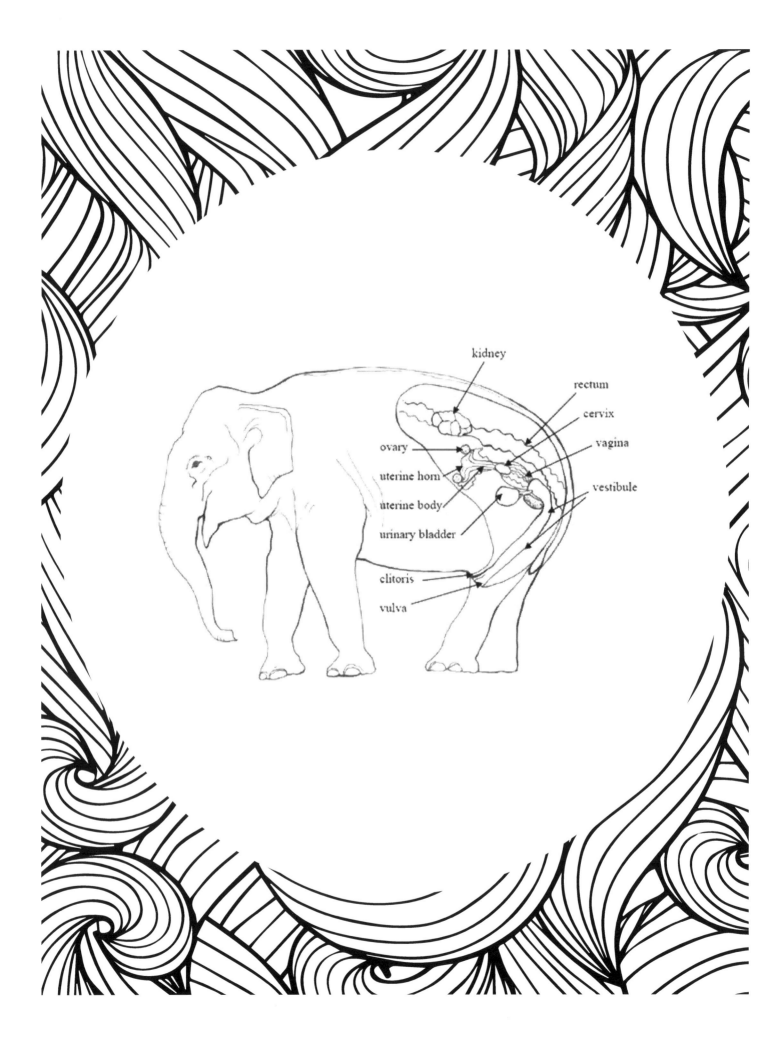

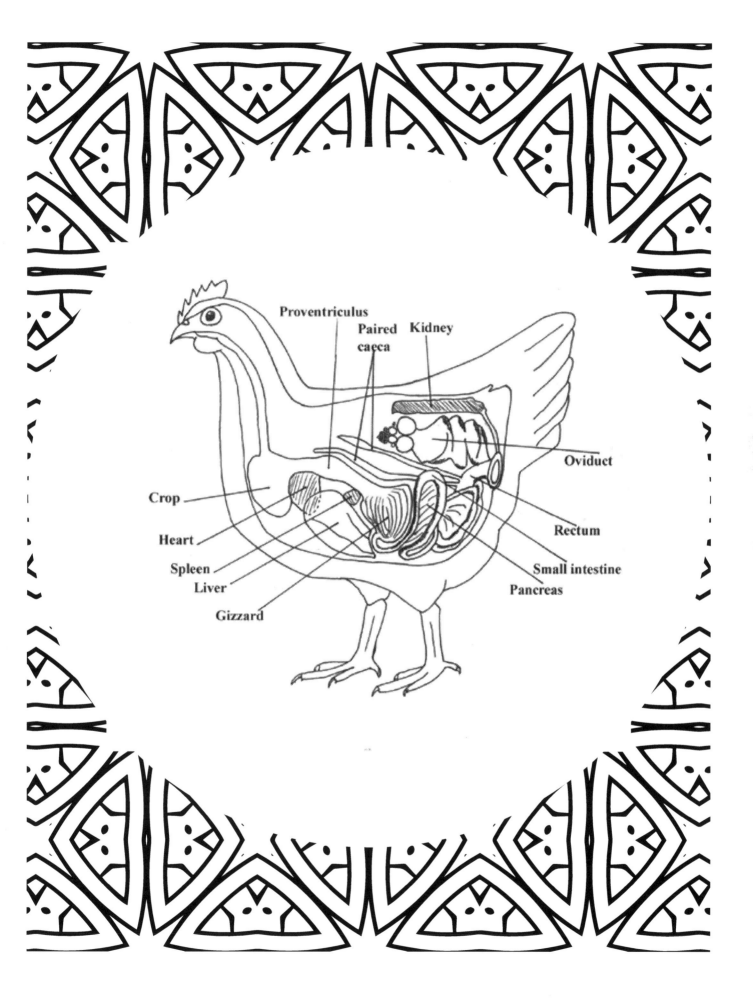

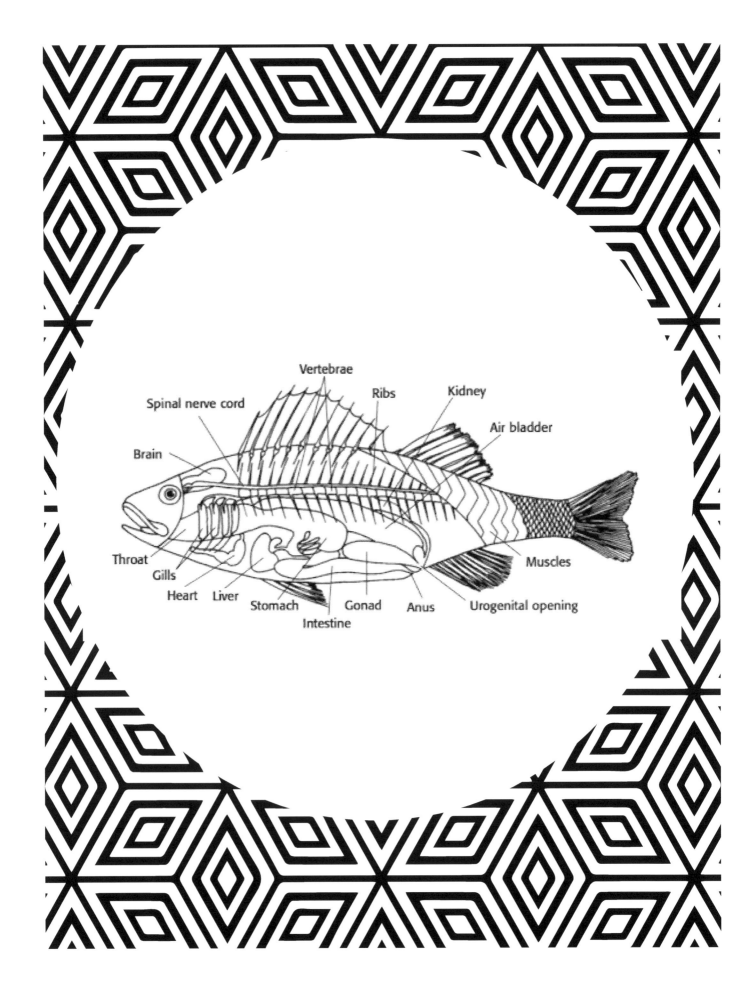

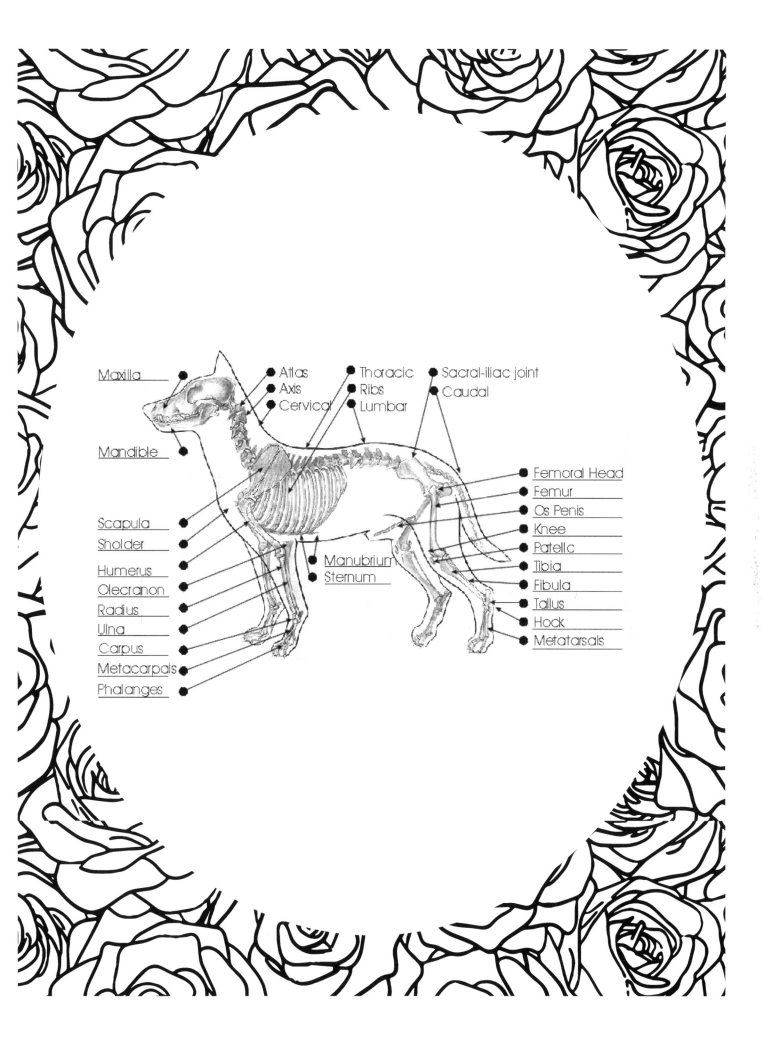

Maxilla

Mandible

Scapula

Sholder

Humerus

Olecranon

Radius

Ulna

Carpus

Metacarpals

Phalanges

Atlas

Axis

Cervical

Manubrium
Sternum

Thoracic

Ribs

Lumbar

Sacral-iliac joint

Caudal

Femoral Head

Femur

Os Penis

Knee

Patellc

Tibia

Fibula

Tallus

Hock

Metatarsals

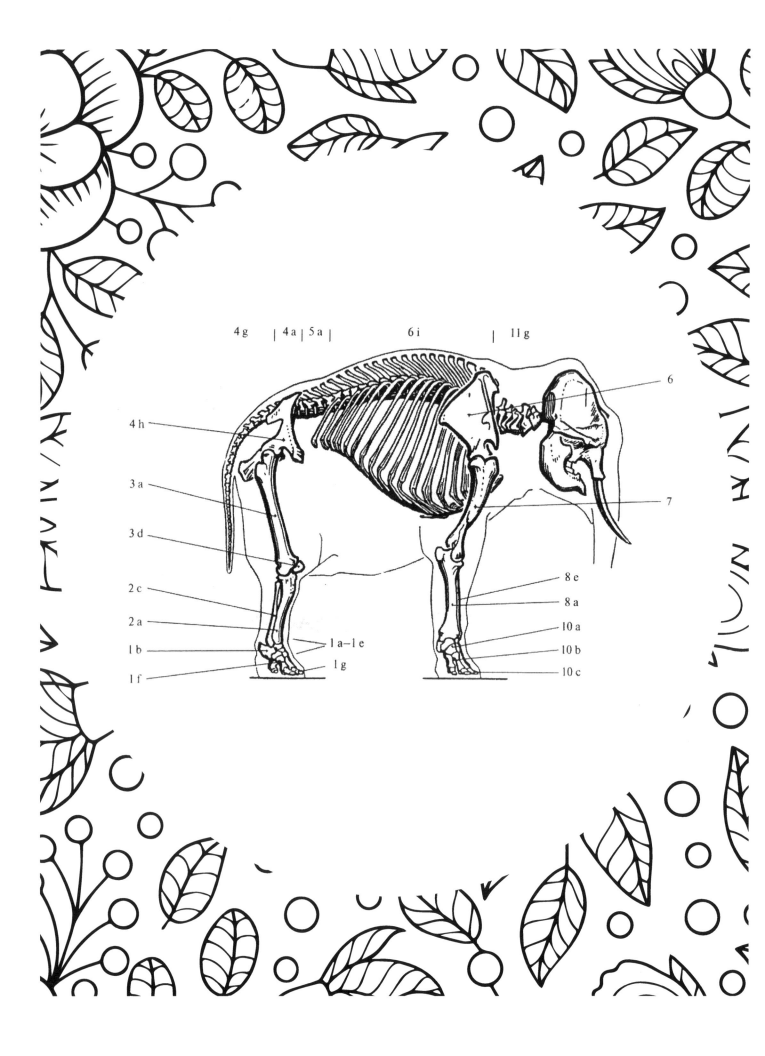

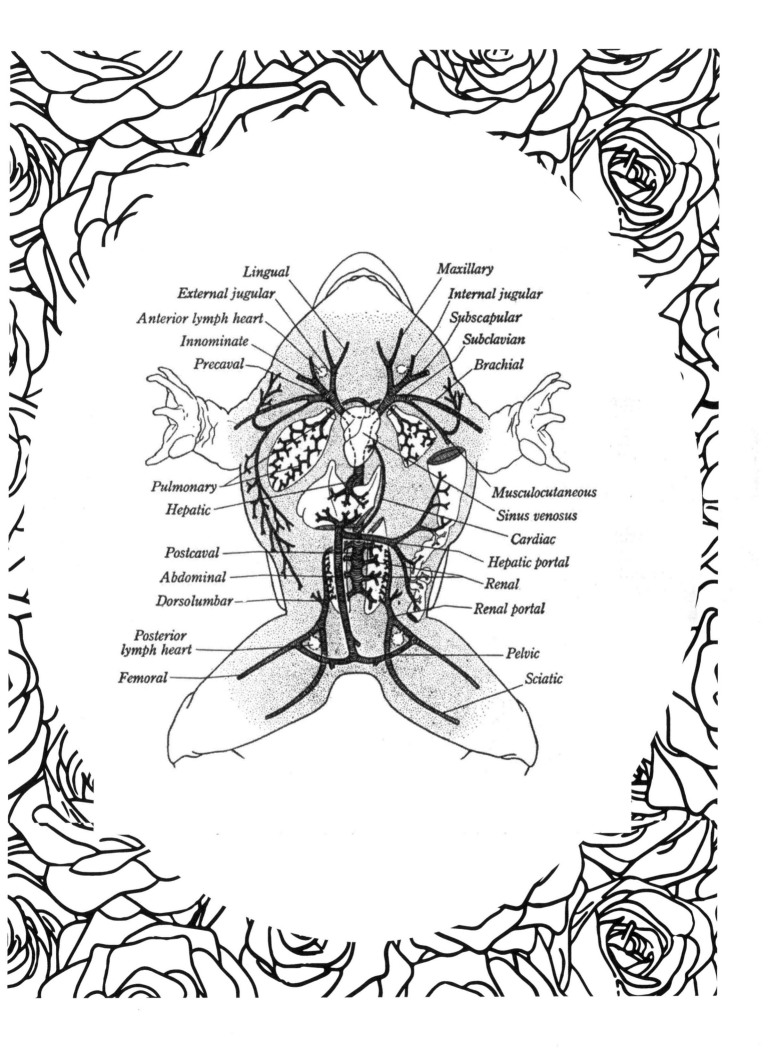

Lingual

Maxillary

External jugular

Internal jugular

Anterior lymph heart

Subscapular

Innominate

Subclavian

Precaval

Brachial

Pulmonary

Musculocutaneous

Hepatic

Sinus venosus

Cardiac

Postcaval

Hepatic portal

Abdominal

Renal

Dorsolumbar

Renal portal

Posterior
lymph heart

Pelvic

Femoral

Sciatic

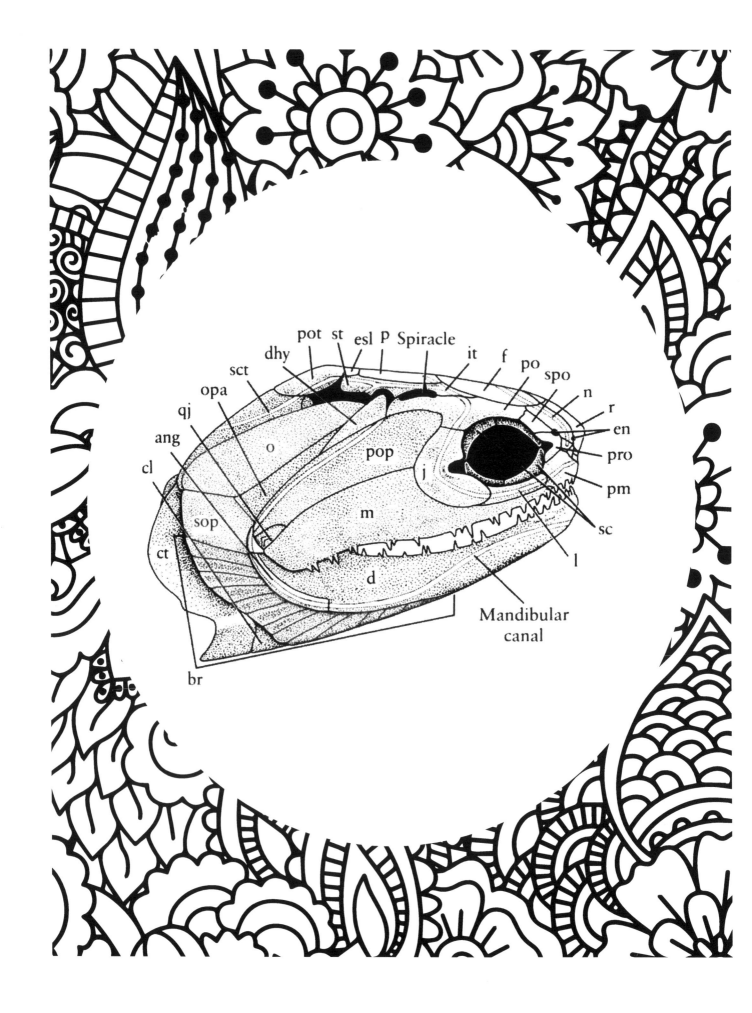

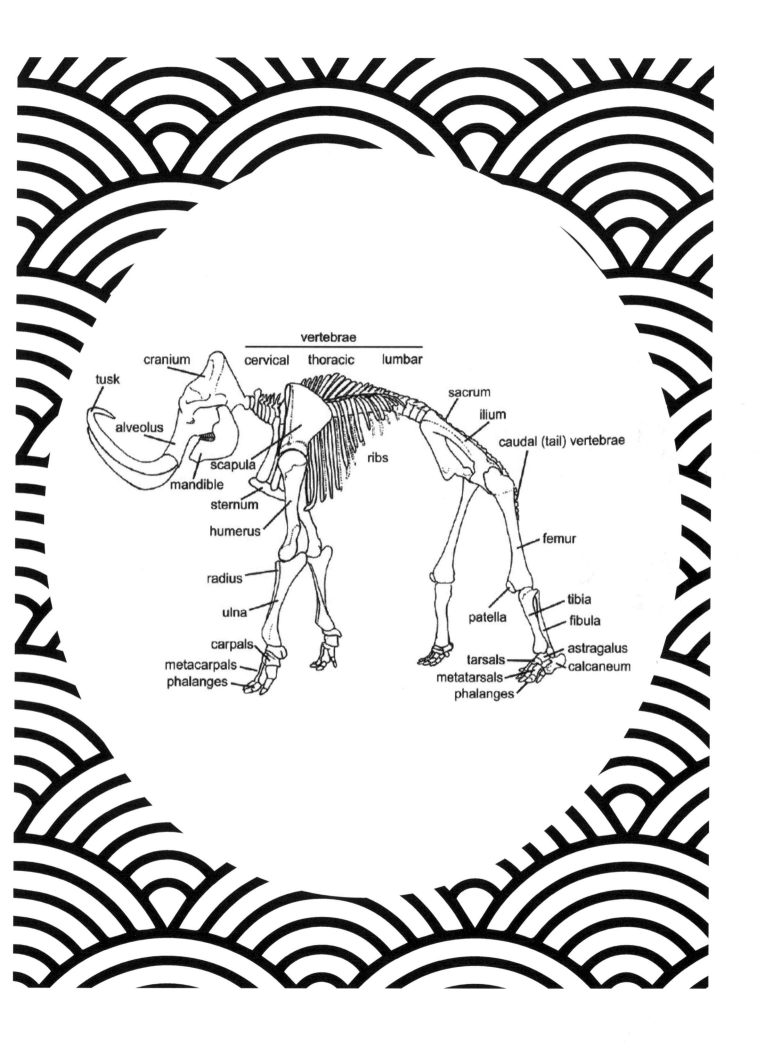

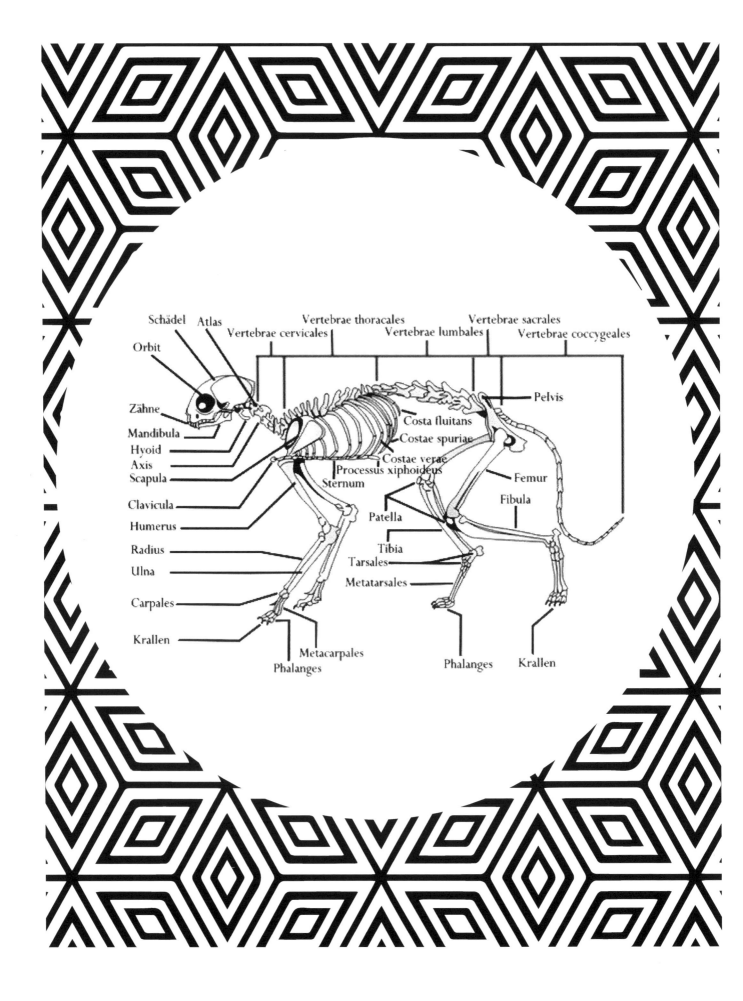

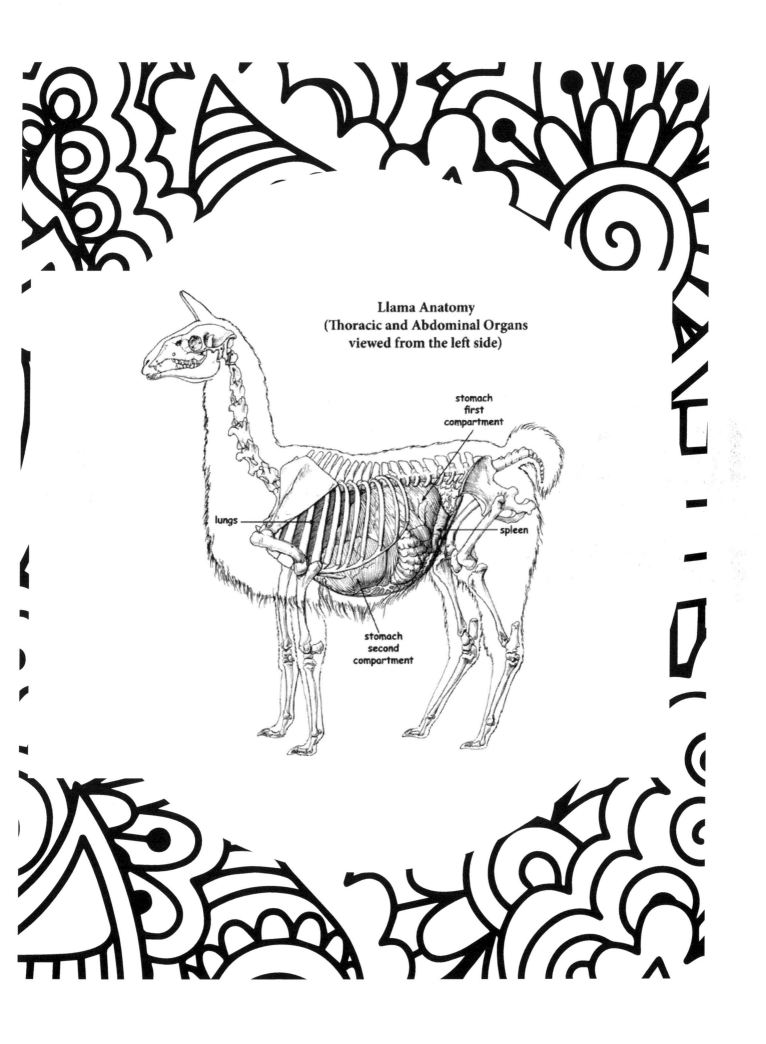

Llama Anatomy
(Thoracic and Abdominal Organs
viewed from the left side)

stomach
first
compartment

lungs

spleen

stomach
second
compartment

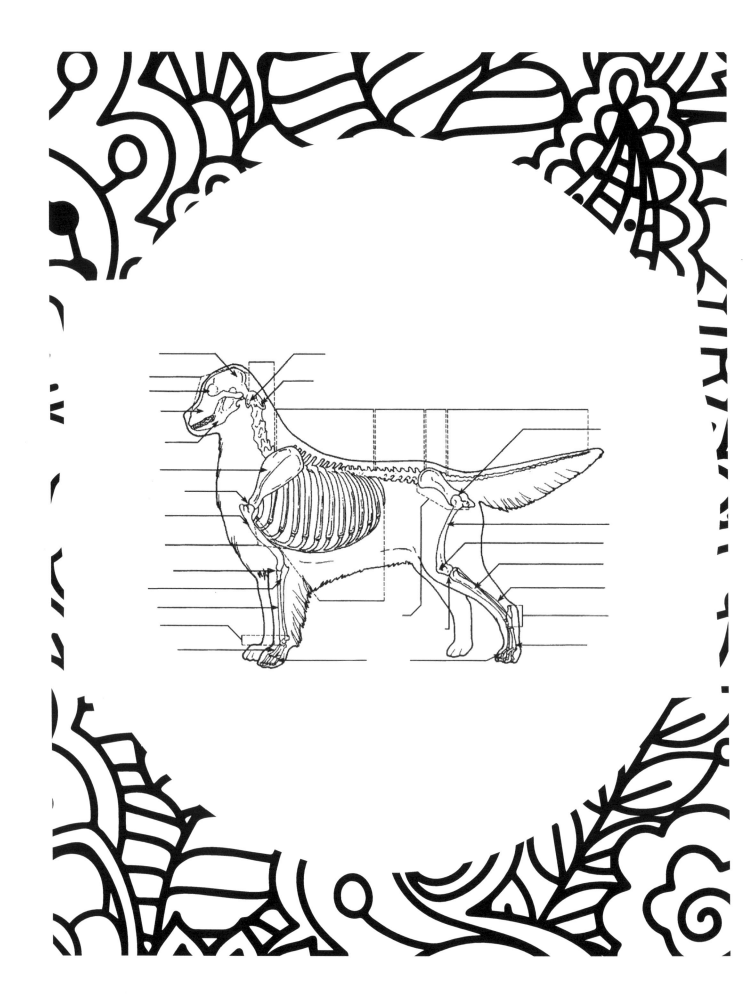

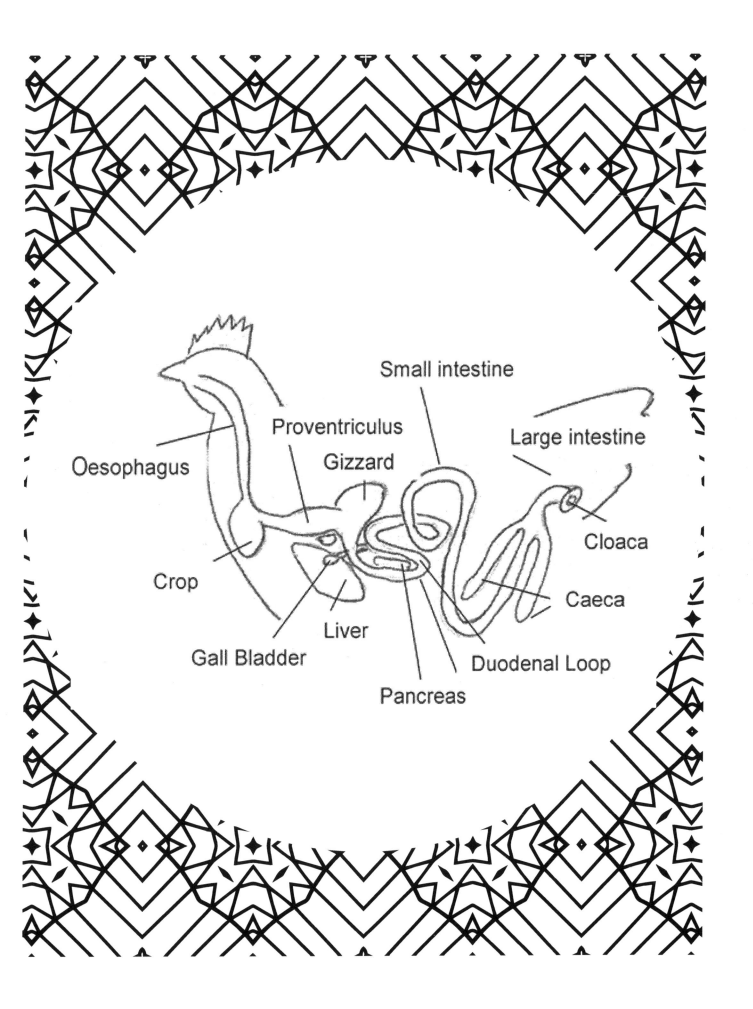

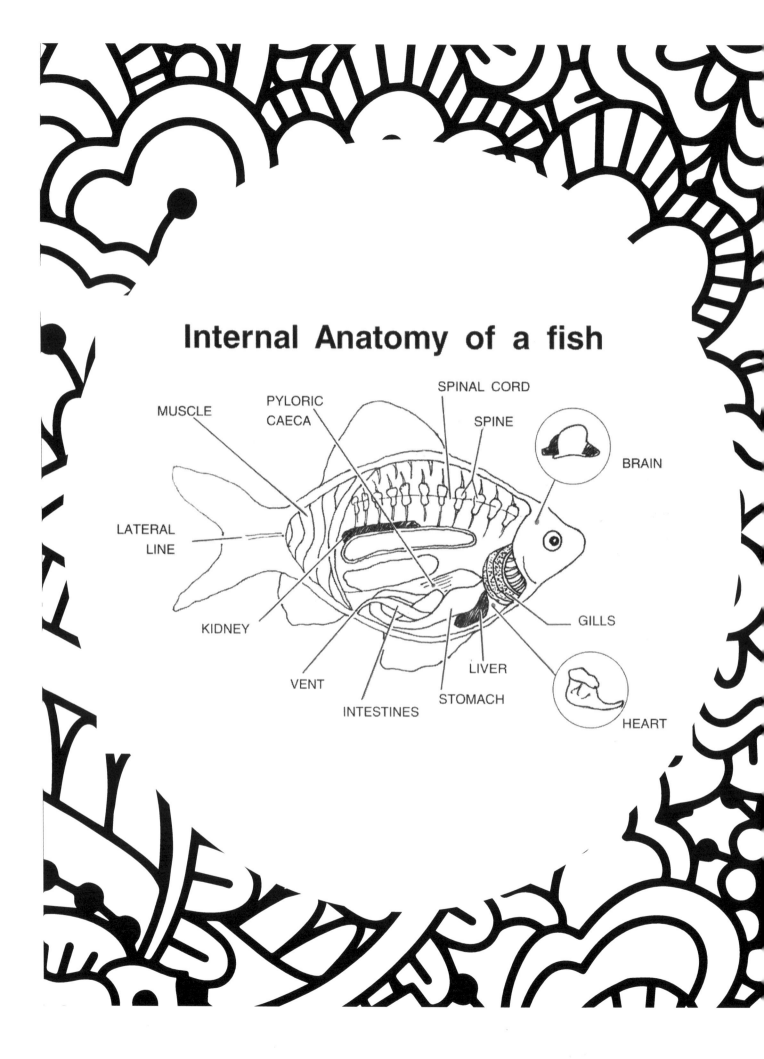

Internal Anatomy of a fish

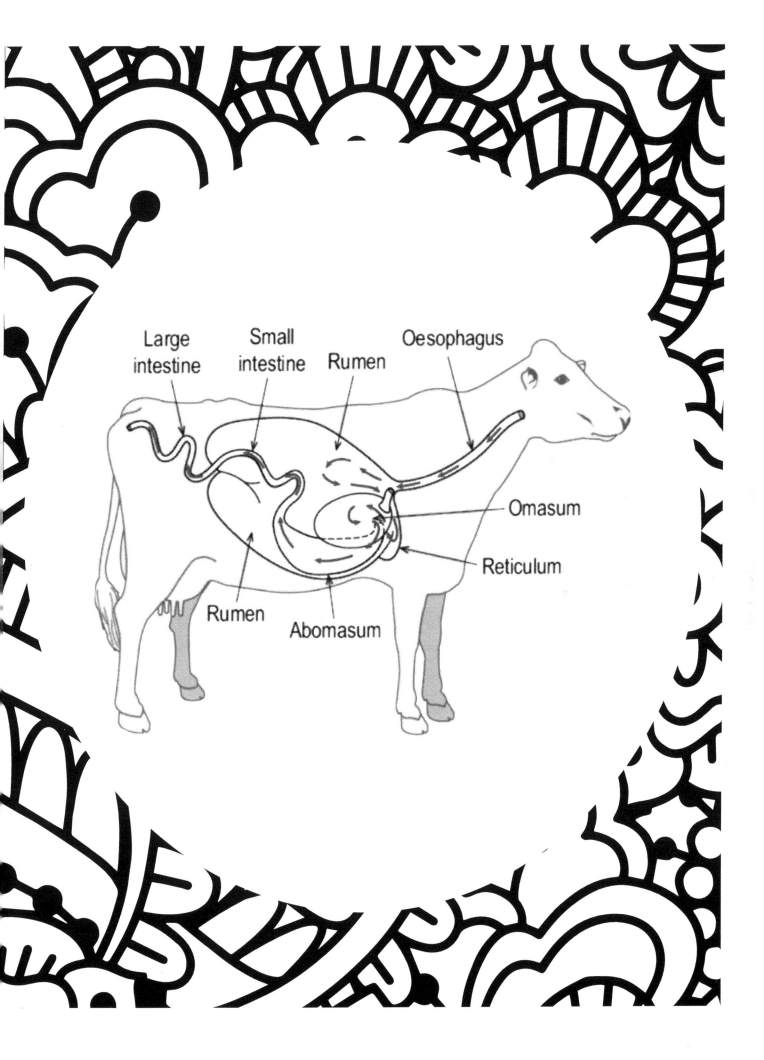

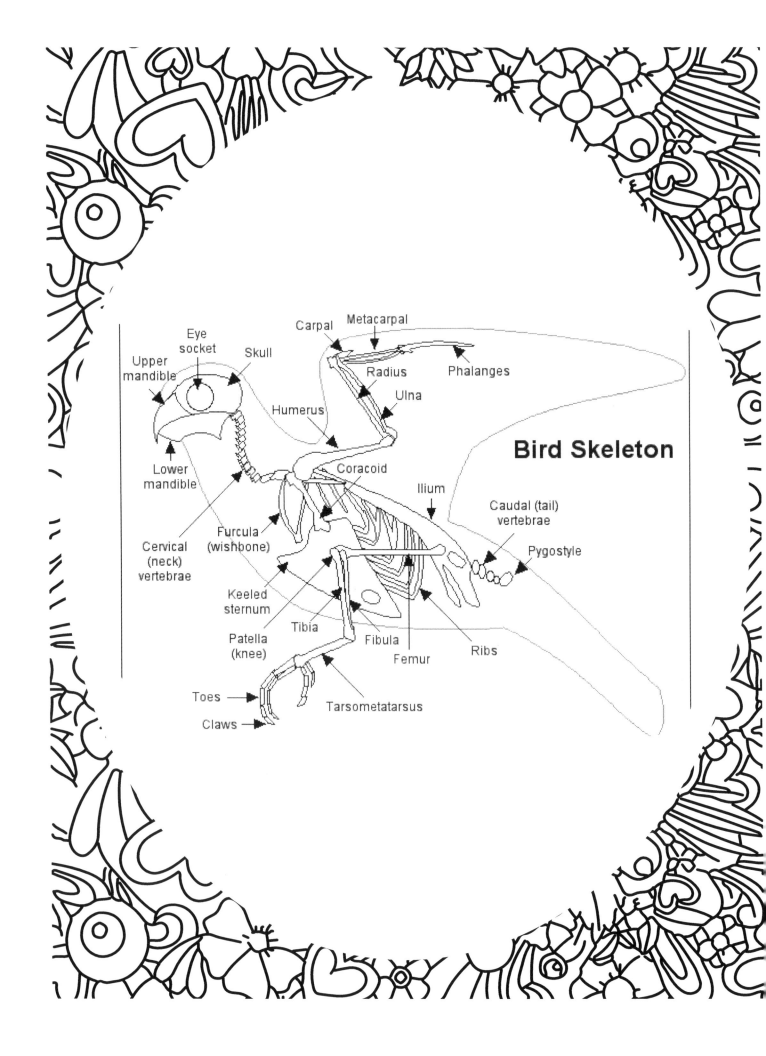

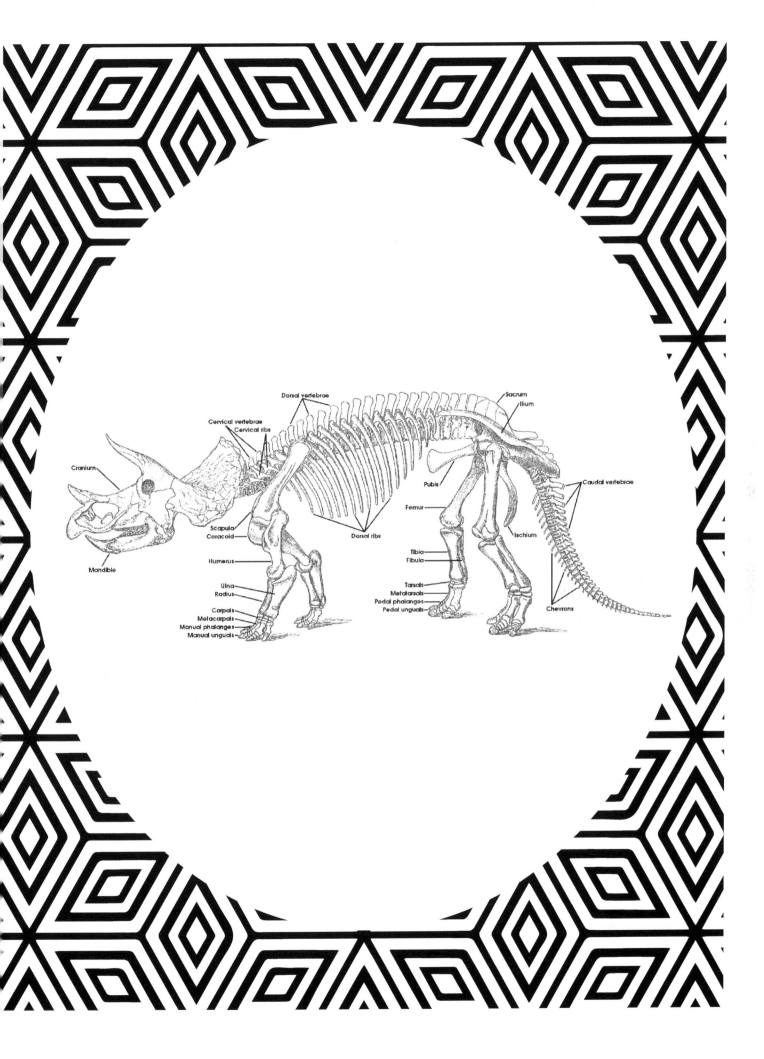

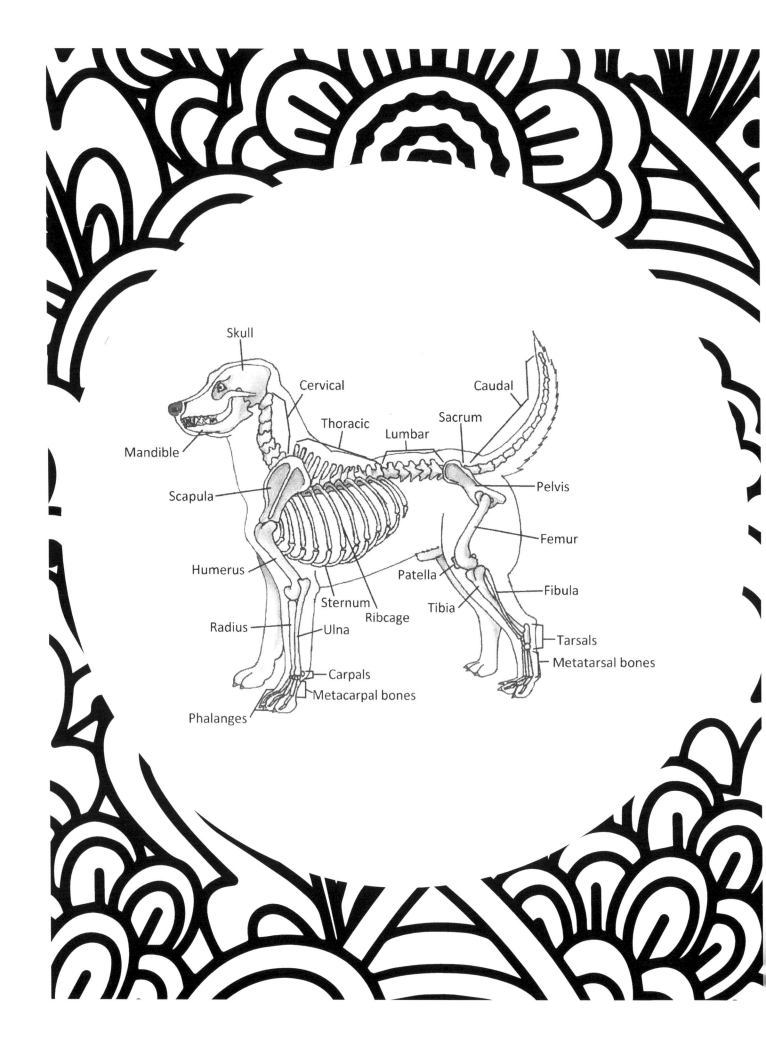

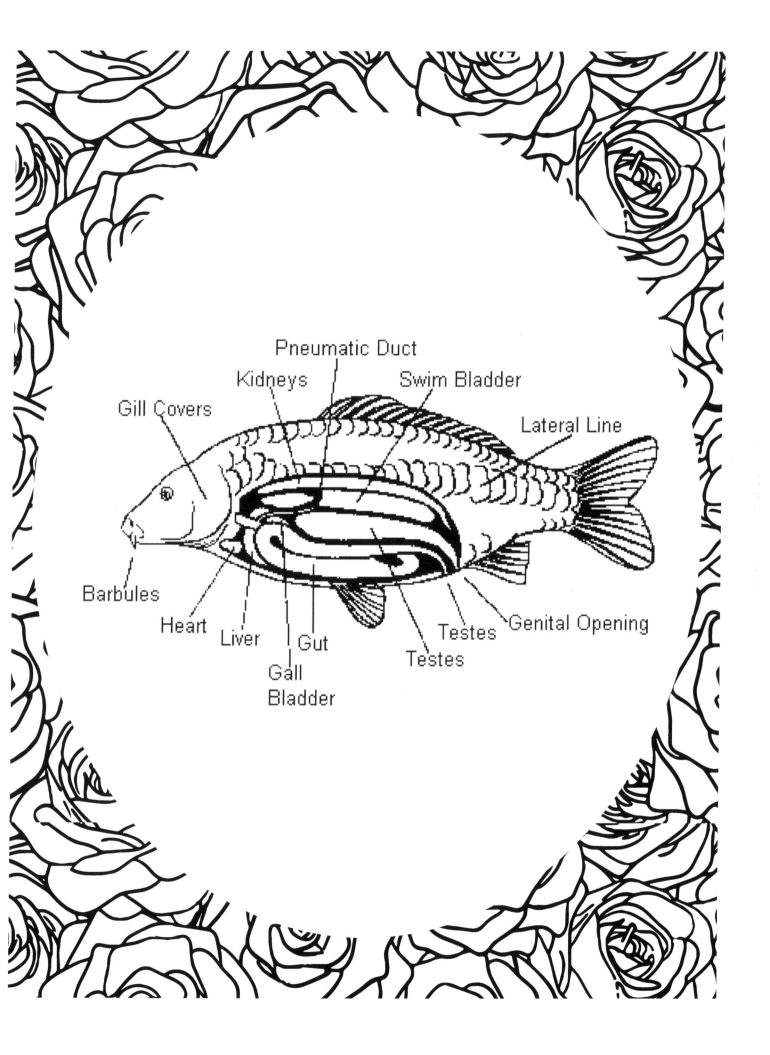

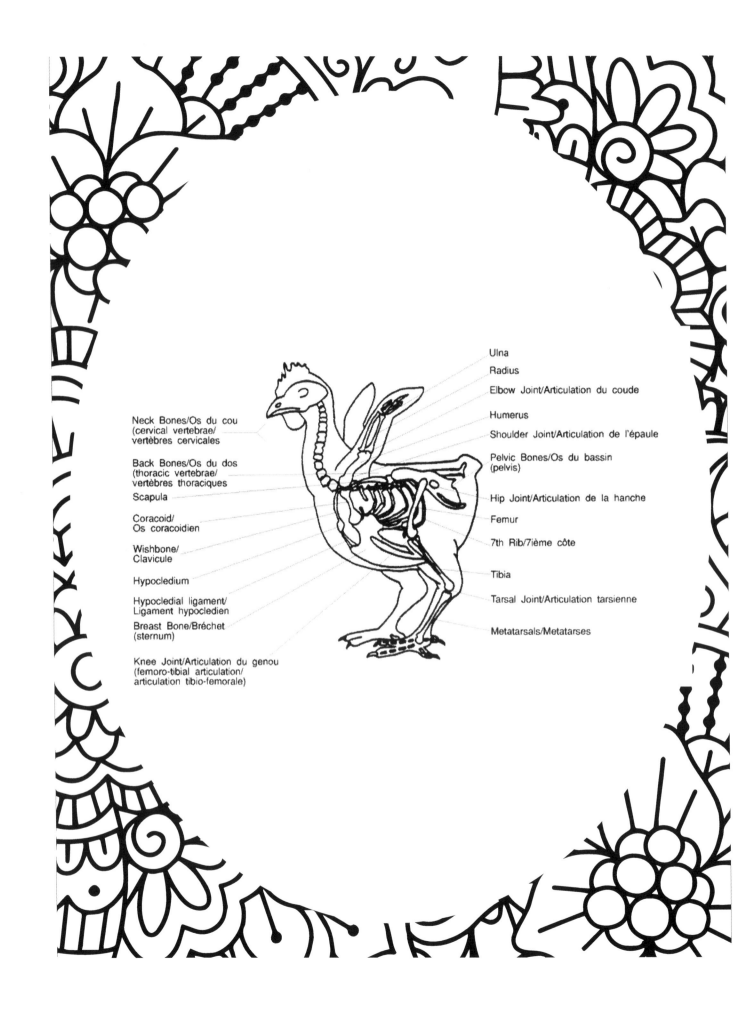

Neck Bones/Os du cou
(cervical vertebrae/
vertèbres cervicales

Back Bones/Os du dos
(thoracic vertebrae/
vertèbres thoraciques

Scapula

Coracoid/
Os coracoidien

Wishbone/
Clavicule

Hypocledium

Hypocledial ligament/
Ligament hypocledien

Breast Bone/Bréchet
(sternum)

Knee Joint/Articulation du genou
(femoro-tibial articulation/
articulation tibio-femorale)

Ulna

Radius

Elbow Joint/Articulation du coude

Humerus

Shoulder Joint/Articulation de l'épaule

Pelvic Bones/Os du bassin
(pelvis)

Hip Joint/Articulation de la hanche

Femur

7th Rib/7ième côte

Tibia

Tarsal Joint/Articulation tarsienne

Metatarsals/Metatarses

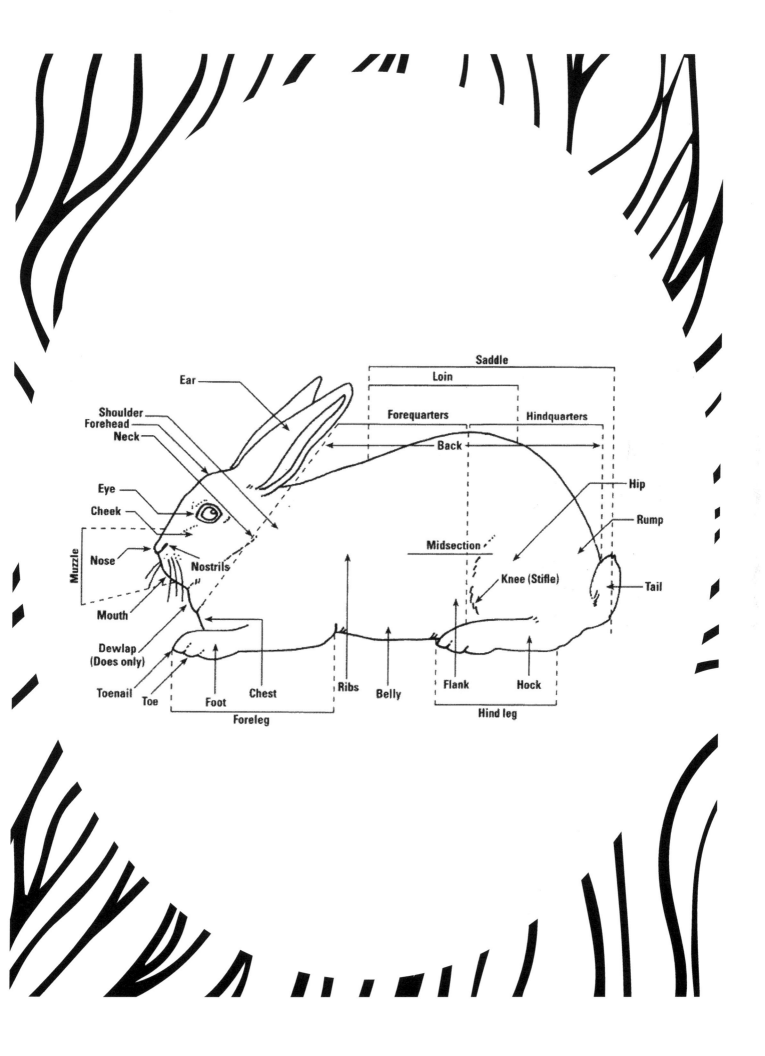

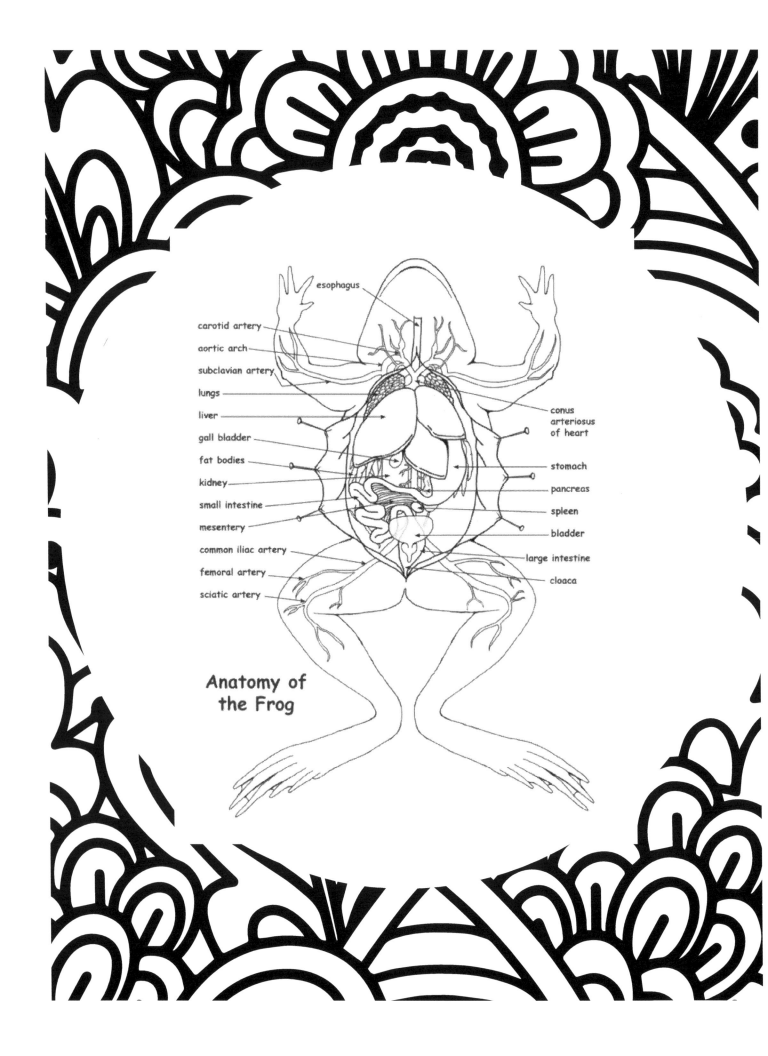

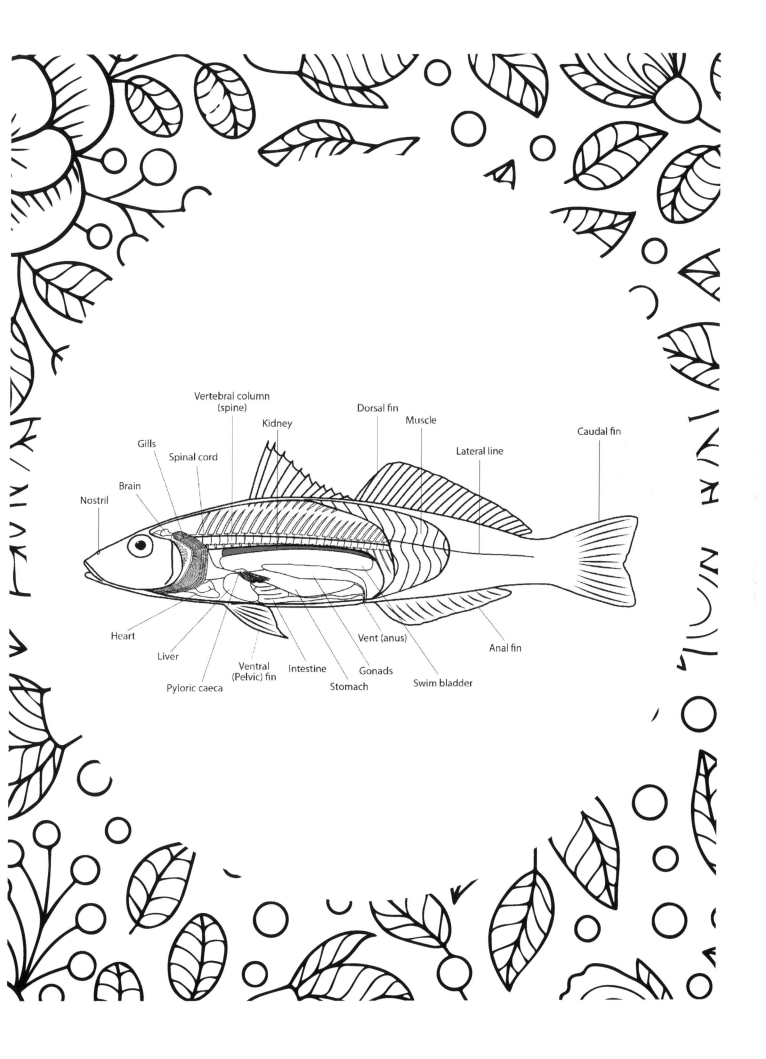

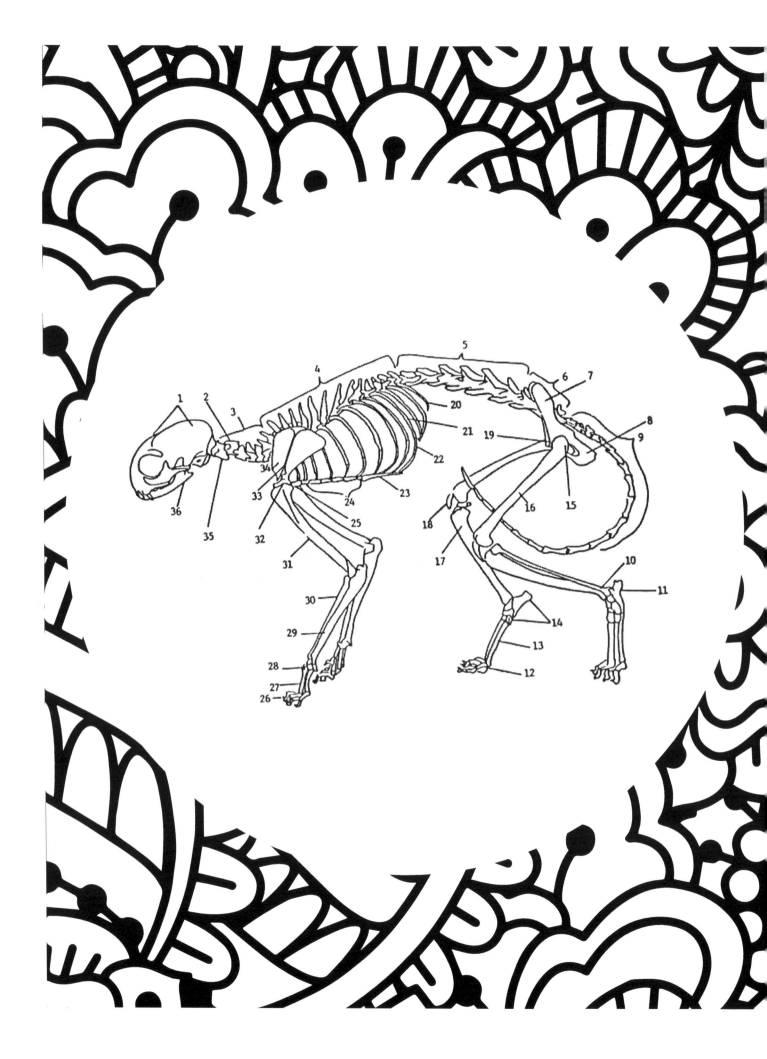

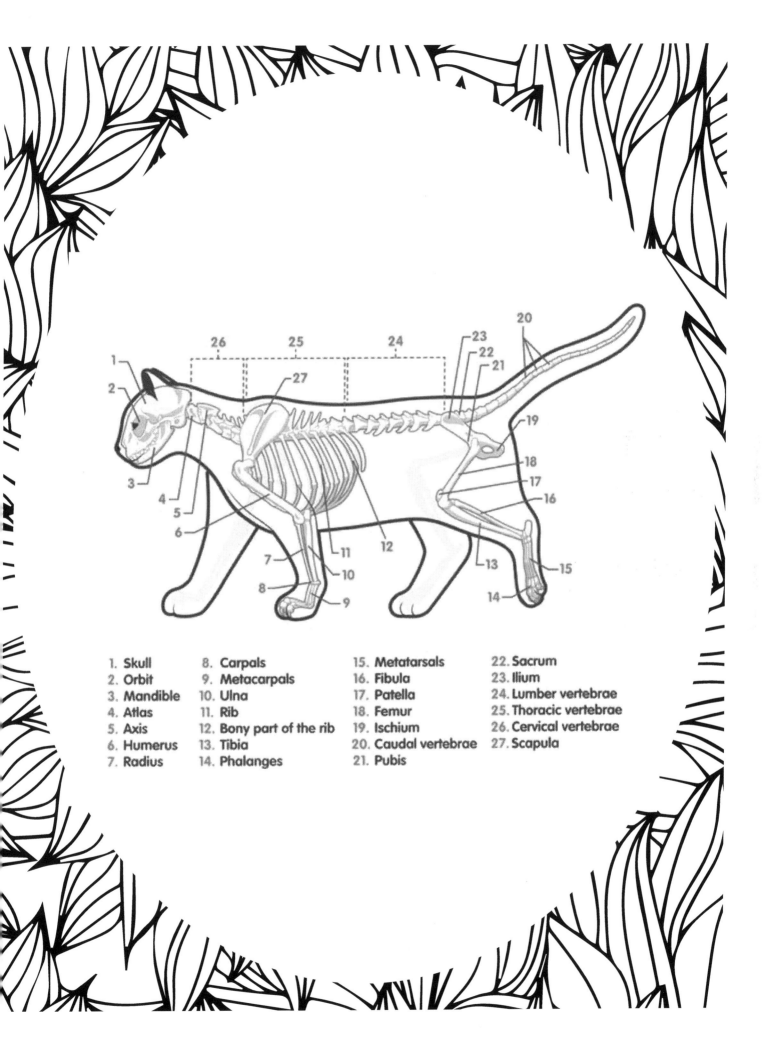

1. Skull
2. Orbit
3. Mandible
4. Atlas
5. Axis
6. Humerus
7. Radius
8. Carpals
9. Metacarpals
10. Ulna
11. Rib
12. Bony part of the rib
13. Tibia
14. Phalanges
15. Metatarsals
16. Fibula
17. Patella
18. Femur
19. Ischium
20. Caudal vertebrae
21. Pubis
22. Sacrum
23. Ilium
24. Lumber vertebrae
25. Thoracic vertebrae
26. Cervical vertebrae
27. Scapula

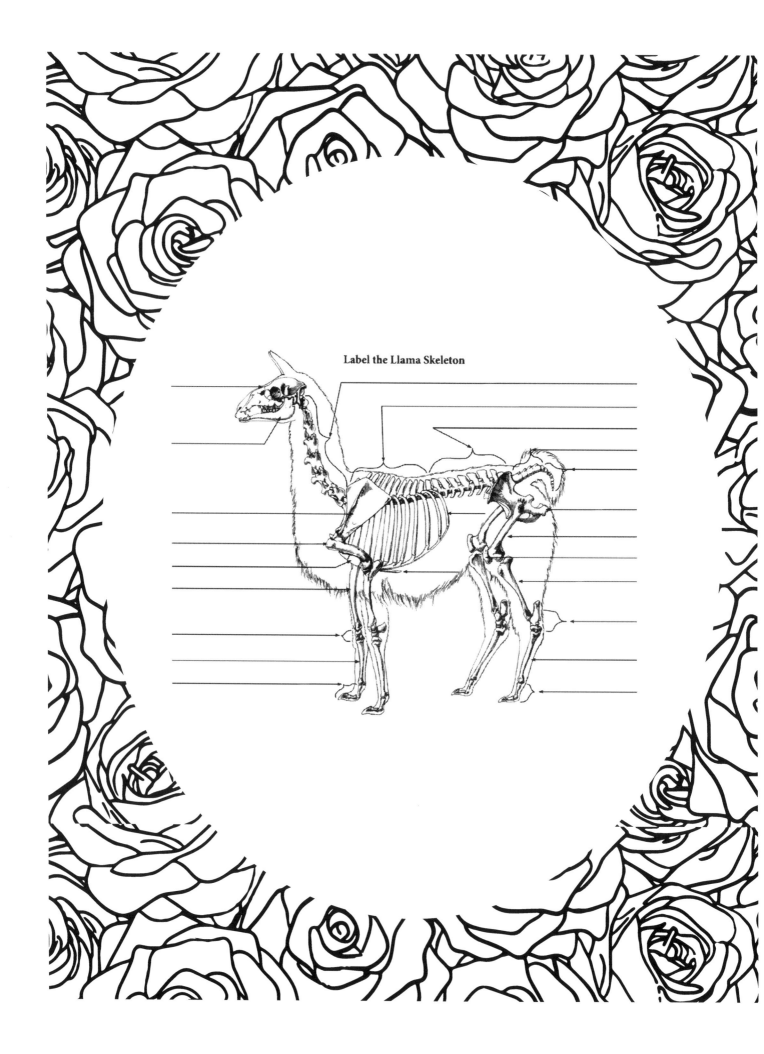

Label the Llama Skeleton

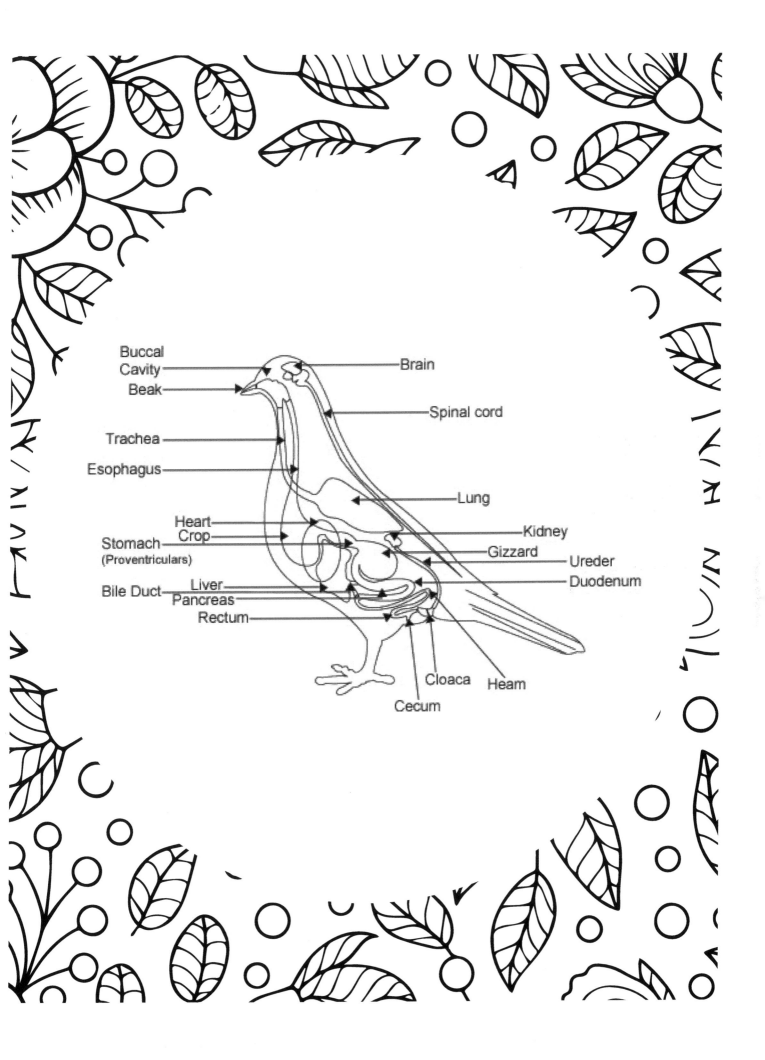

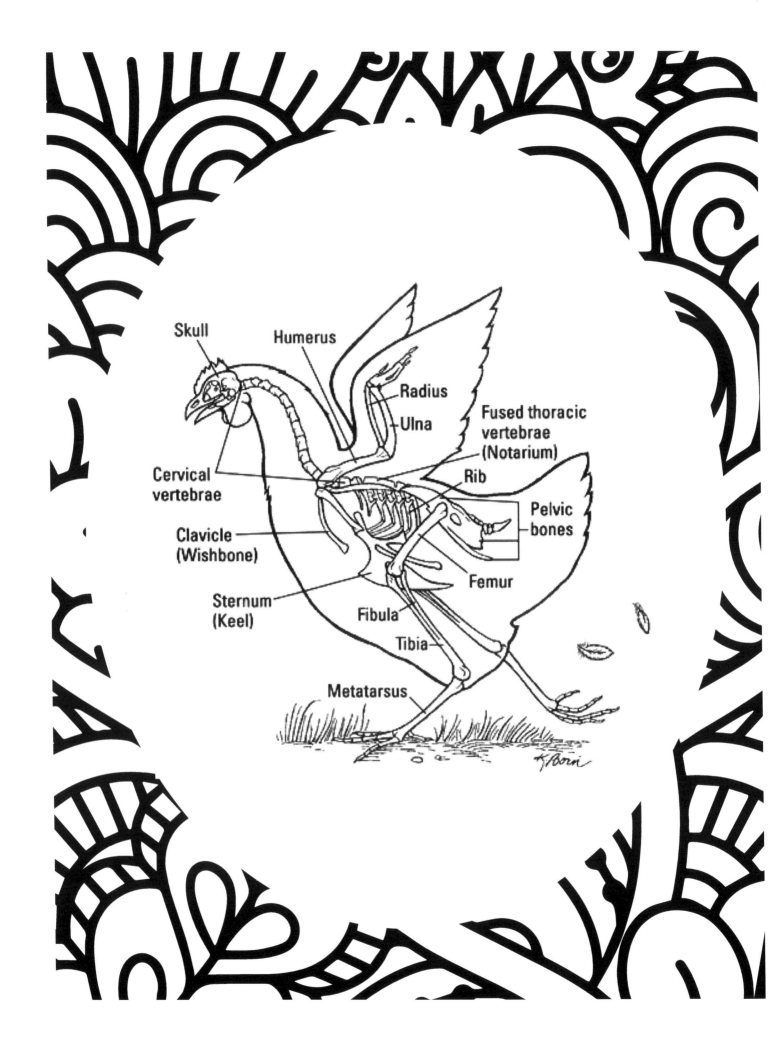

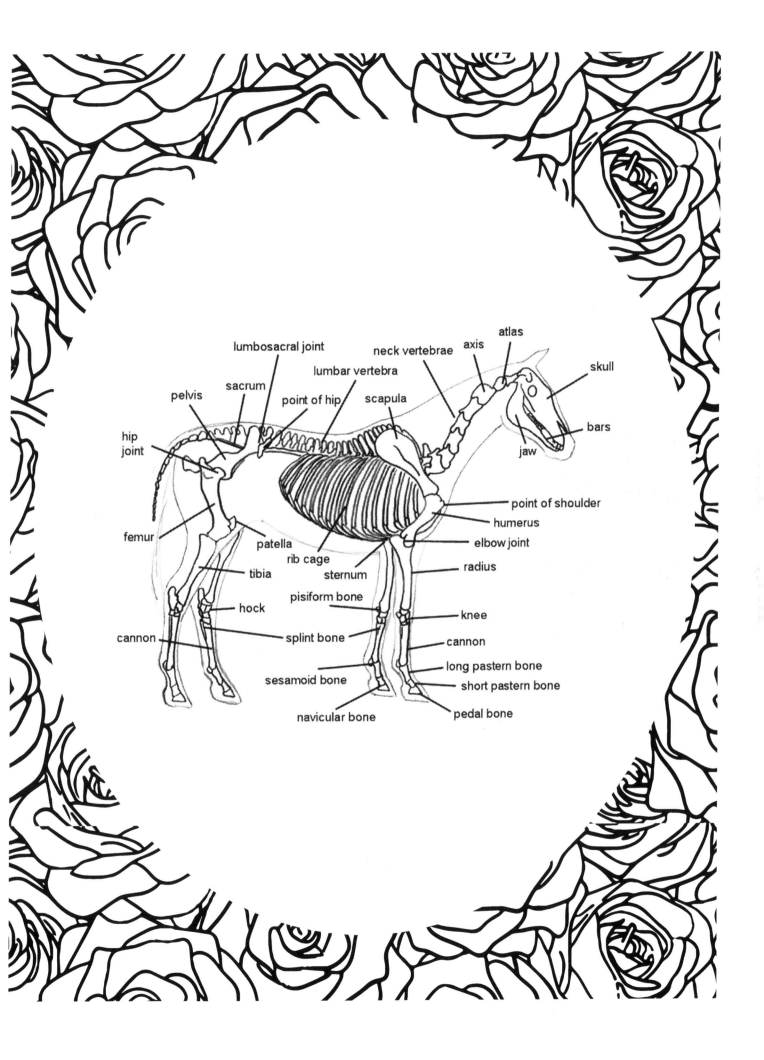

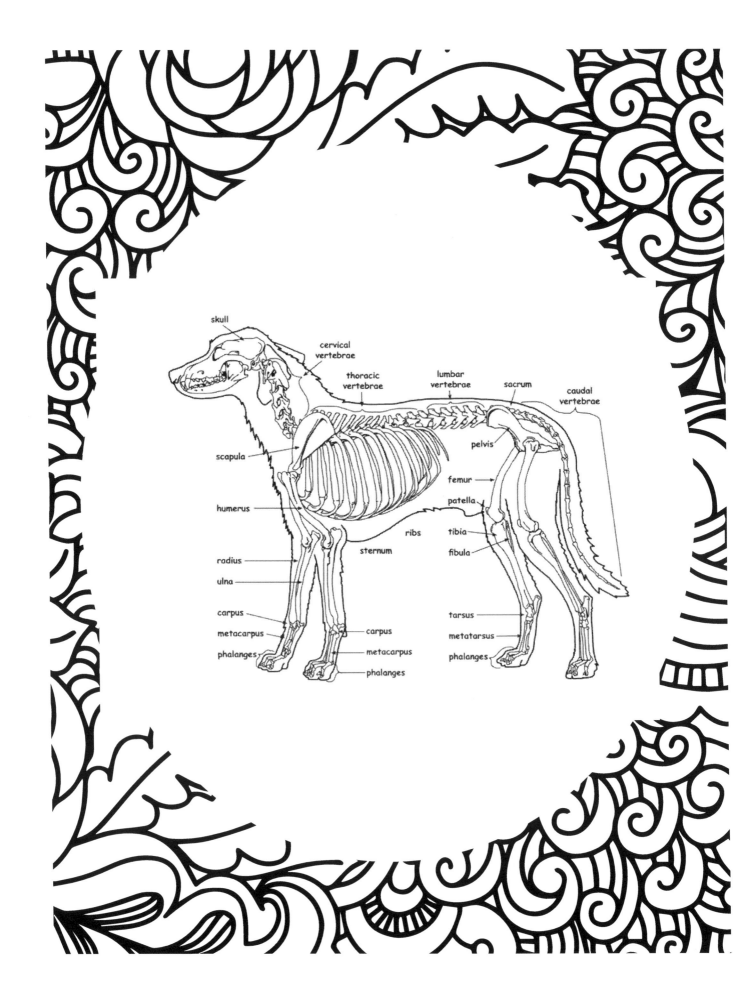

Printed in Great Britain
by Amazon

65679646R00029